The Green Smoothie Challenge

Companion

by

Maria Rippo

thegreensmoothiechallenge.com

WisdomWithinPublishing.com

Columbus Ohio

Book cover and layout design by Rachel Hoffmann, Orange Peel Design

Published by Be Wellthy, Inc., Seattle, WA and WisdomWithinPublishing.com, Columbus, OH

For publisher permission, please contact maria@thegreensmoothiechallenge.com

Disclaimer:

The Green Smoothie Challenge Companion has been written for informational purposes only and is in no way intended as medical advice, a substitute for medical counseling, or as a treatment/ cure for any disease or health condition nor should it be interpreted as such. Be Wellthy, Inc. and its publishers are not medical doctors, nor is this document to be considered, in any way, medical advice. Consequently, this information is provided in an "as-is" basis and is for informational purposes only. The reader assumes all risks associated directly or indirectly from the use, non-use or misuse of this information. BE WELLTHY INC. EXPRESSLY DISCLAIMS ALL EXPRESS OR IMPLIED WARRANTIES, INCLUDING, WITHOUT LIMITATION, THE IMPLIED WARRANTIES OF MERCHANTABILITY, FITNESS FOR A PARTICULAR PURPOSE AND NON-INFRINGEMENT, AND FURTHER, BECAUSE BE WELLTHY, INC., ITS OFFICERS, DIRECTORS AND/OR EMPLOYEES ARE NOT DOCTORS, THEY DO NOT PROVIDE, AND EXPRESSLY DISCLAIM, ALL WARRANTIES, EXPRESS OF IMPLIED, AND ALL OBLIGATIONS OR LIABILITIES FOR DAMAGES ARISING OUT OF OR IN CONNECTION WITH THE USE OR MISUSE OF ANY SUGGESTIONS OR PROCEDURES PUBLISHED IN THIS WORK. Be Wellthy, Inc. encourages you to always work with a qualified health professional before making any changes to your diet, prescription drug use, lifestyle or exercise program.

Bold Links: Throughout the book, you will find words, book titles and other text shown in bold type. In the upcoming digital version of this book, those will be hyperlinks. For the purpose of the printed book, a list of general links has been provided at the end of the book. For specific product links and to download your quick reference guide and 10 day transformation calendar visit **http://www.mariarippo.com/your-green-smoothie-challenge-tool-kit.html**

DEDICATION

This guide is dedicated to Tobin, who has always encouraged me to pursue my passion of practicing natural health and who is my biggest fan. To my children who bring me laughter, endless amounts of joy, challenge me daily and give an honest critique of my healthy food creations. To my family and friends who are an unending source of love and encouragement. To Rachel Rosales who caught my vision and without whom The Green Smoothie Challenge may still be just an idea. To all the amazing raw-food chefs and teachers who have graciously shared their recipes and who inspire me daily. To Victoria Boutenko, for her kindness in sharing her discoveries with the world. And mostly, to the Creator who has opened every door to make this project possible.

CONTENTS

Let thy food be thy medicine, and thy medicine be thy food. – Hippocrates, the father of modern-day medicine.

FOREWORD

The Green Smoothie Challenge is a uniquely simple and healthful tool for anybody. Maria Rippo is introducing her readers to the healthiest beverage that anyone can quickly prepare in their own kitchen. They can embrace the entire week of living solely on green smoothies or add a green drink here and there. This book allows everyone to create their personal Green Smoothie Challenge and benefit from it. I have witnessed countless people becoming healthier and younger from adding green smoothies to their food regimen.

Most people are amazed by the pleasant taste of green smoothies. At the same time, green smoothies are among the healthiest foods available to us. Greens are the only living thing in the world that can transform sunshine into food that all creatures can consume. Chlorophyll is a miraculous substance as it is in essence liquefied sunshine. That is why regular consumption of green smoothies can help with many different health problems.

With this book, Maria Rippo is reaching out to hundreds and thousands of people with a very healthful and helpful message. Dear friends, enjoy your Green Smoothie Challenge and pass it on to others!

Victoria Boutenko

Author of *Green for Life* and *Green Smoothie Revolution*

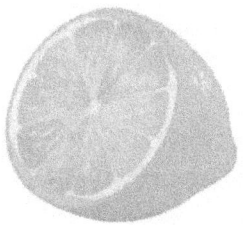

ABOUT THE AUTHOR

Carefree, but...

I grew up in the sunny land of San Diego, California. I spent many hours on the beach, enjoying all the outdoor activities that fresh air, sunshine, and wide-open land affords. Growing up, I was actively involved in sports such as softball, field hockey, competitive gymnastics and horseback riding. I loved swimming and being outside as much as possible. I thought I was a fairly healthy child but as I have worked through a myriad of health issues in my adult life, I see that my struggles started when I was young.

I was born jaundiced. I was inflicted with many ear infections resulting in the use of antibiotics. I had a difficult time paying attention in school. I never remember feeling great; my stomach usually hurt. I was an extremely picky eater, totally obsessed with junk food and sugar. I would go to my friends' houses after school just so I could get my sugar fix! When I visited my grandma and grandpa, my first question was, "What's for dessert?" I remember stealing candy from the store once, when I was in Kindergarten.

As the story goes, I was stubborn from the start. Much to my dismay, my mother did not allow any junk food in our home which made me all the more ravenous to eat as much of it as I could whenever the opportunity presented itself. I was very thin as a child and did not particularly thrive. According to my mom, at two years old, I would only eat about ten foods. The doctor said I was on the verge of being malnourished because I simply refused to eat (can you say stubborn?)!

Catching the Natural Health Fever

While still in college, I became aware that I felt utterly exhausted; much more than I knew I ought to feel at that age. That's when a good friend introduced me to the ideas of fresh juice fasting and living foods. This was a welcome break from the diet of a college student and made a huge difference in how I felt. My energy exploded. My skin cleared up. I released all my extra weight. My experience of adding these new foods to my diet was so life changing that I became an avid researcher of alternative medicine and natural health. Meeting people cured through natural means from diseases such as cancer and AIDS fascinated me and instilled in me a great passion for this subject. I've had a keen interest in natural health for over twenty years now.

I received my BA from Oregon State University. While there, I found myself mostly alone in my quest for optimum health. As I began my new journey, I ate healthy much of the time. However, I never overcame my sugar and junk food addiction completely. I would eat really well and then go to the grocery store and buy a pint of chocolate chip cookie dough ice cream and a large bag of peanut butter M&M's® and eat all of it in one sitting. I didn't know how to live in moderation with mindfulness and gratitude at the center of my eating choices. When feeling particularly out of control, I would use fresh juice fasting as a means to get back on track and it worked wonders for me. It felt so freeing to take a break from all the foods that had a hold on me. My mind would clear up and I became motivated and inspired. But then I would slide back into the place where I felt out of control towards my cravings, giving in and starting the cycle over again. It seemed that sugar and junk food called my name relentlessly. I now realize that a physiological dopamine response is triggered in the brain when one ingests processed foods that contain a combination of sugar, fat and salt. These foods "change the biological circuitry of our brains." My cravings for these foods were physiological; my brain was asking to have its pleasure center stimulated. But, they were also emotional in nature because of their ability to numb deep-seated pain that I didn't even know existed!

Food is Good Medicine. Or is it?

I was in my thirties before I was also able to see that I had become an emotional eater. (It is thought that 70% of us are emotional eaters.) I ate foods I vowed not to eat instead of realizing that my cravings were messengers showing me areas of life that felt empty. I was numbing myself with food. I was self-medicating because I had not learned how to process the hurts, stresses, frustrations and sorrows that are a normal part of this earthly existence. Although I ate healthy, I still had a secret love affair with sugar and chocolate. I lived in an unhealthy cycle of overeating or making food choices that I knew would not promote optimal health and then hating myself for it and going into a cycle of restriction.

The Scale Slave

I lived this yo-yo for many years, although knowing how to eat healthfully helped me maintain a decent weight. I was a slave to the scale. The number it revealed each day would dictate my mood. I ate healthy all week and then binged on weekends. This, along with my natural inclination to stuff my emotions inside me, hoping to never feel them, finally caught up with me in the form of big health challenges, namely chronic fatigue and manic depression.

---

[1] Kessler, David A., The End of Overeating: Controlling the Insatiable American Appetite, Rodale Inc., New York, NY, 2009.

The Gift of Losing Everything

When my fourth child was eighteen months old, my dear father-in-law passed very suddenly. Six weeks later, my dad had a massive stroke. After these devastating experiences, we went bankrupt and lost our home. My marriage relationship suffered greatly. What followed was my wake-up call. I got eczema all over both eyes, of all places. I had never had skin issues before. I also noticed that the lines between my eyebrows were deepening. I felt I was becoming ugly. I hated my husband, my life. I was mad at God and the world for the lot I had been given. I grew up thinking I would live *the life,* and that was not happening. I thought it was *the life* that would make me happy, the happily-ever-after story. I wanted glass slippers! But, in reality, I was resisting life. I knew no other way. Losing everything woke me up to the misery that had already existed in me. I knew I could not go on this way. I knew I needed help!

The End of My Self-Hatred

This was the beginning of my journey into true healing. I began to heal the wounds from childhood with a therapist and holistic coach, focusing on learning self-compassion and healed negative experiences I had as a young girl. I learned how to nurture and have reverence for myself instead of grasping for it from outside sources.

I also began my adventure of healing my physical body through nourishing foods. As I became physically stronger, I was able to work at a deeper level on my emotional wellbeing. A few times I slipped for a few weeks and boy, did it bring me back down. I have found that if I eat foods that are part of the Standard American Diet (SAD), I become a hormonal basket case, my skin breaks out, my energy takes a hike, my mood dives, my food cravings return, my mind gets foggy and cluttered, I become uninspired, and my pants get smaller. Some food is like poison to my system. It literally changes who I am, and I am thankful to say that I have come to the point where I have no interest in allowing those foods to make me feel that way.

As I felt better and changed my thinking patterns, I began to see my own value. I imagined myself fully healthy. I began to hear my thoughts and change them from being habitually negative, to being more proactive and empowering rather than destructive. I began to see my food cravings as powerful messengers that were a catalyst for my growth and transformation rather than a sign I was somehow defective. It was during this time of healing that I learned about green smoothies from Victoria Boutenko. They were a lifesaver for me because of their affordability, simplicity and health-providing miraculous nature. As I began to drink them, I noticed my skin softened and hydrated, my energy levels skyrocketed and my overall ability to deal with life in a healthy manner improved.

I Loved Myself No Matter How Much I Weighed

As I felt better and began to see my own unique gifts and to use those gifts, and as I changed my focus from hiding from all my ways of self-sabotage and punishment to self-compassion and understanding, I began to have more space in my life to bless others with my gifts, and to live in my truth. I was able to change my relationship with food for good. It was when I learned to be curious, rather than self-judging, that I began to see very positive changes. I learned to find ways to honor myself no matter how much I weighed and show gratitude to my body for all the ways it serves me and works so hard in ways I don't even understand; i.e. my heart beats without me doing anything, my lungs take in air even while I sleep. I learned to find compassion for myself if I slipped up. I stopped telling myself that I couldn't eat this or that, and I began adding in healthy foods to the point that I just didn't want the other options. I realized that my struggles with food and fat were powerful messengers to show me the parts of my life that were imbalanced. As I healed on an emotional level and began to learn healthy limits and boundaries and how to live from my truth, my challenges with food began to disappear naturally. One by one, I let the habits that did not serve my best interests, go. Little by little, I uncovered my buried emotions. I wanted to be kind to myself. I learned how to feel my feelings. I realized that holding onto resentment was like me drinking poison and expecting the other person to die. I began to let go of my bitterness and realized that the only person whom I was hurting was me. I stopped trying so hard to be something other than I was and began unfolding who I was created to be and loving that person. I finally got that trying to lose weight was futile because weight was a symptom and not the issue.

Vibrant Health is a Journey

As I healed and found my inner fire igniting, I was given the amazing gift of partnering with others on their journey towards health. I introduced many people to green smoothies and helped them go on ten-day green smoothie cleanses – letting go of all the junk and addictive foods for ten short days. The results were astounding, as you will read in the testimonials that follow.

An important truth I have learned along the way is that vibrant health is a journey. It is a destination that we never stop working towards. Health is never about a number on that insignificant, mood-dictating machine we call a scale. That number can do more damage than good for many of us. When I put my focus on becoming a wholly well person, that number no longer mattered to me. I put my scale in a place where I don't even see it and I no longer weigh myself. My body has found its optimal weight and stays there.

My Family

I am married to Tobin, whom I met at the lively young age of fourteen. We have introduced four beautiful, laughter-filled children to this world through natural home births. Our children have rarely had need of doctor visits, and have avoided any use of conventional medications such as antibiotics and the like. Although we do not claim to feed these youthful beings perfectly, they have been raised on a largely whole and living-foods diet. All of them have experienced much better health than my husband or I did as children. They currently regularly beg me for my delectable raw and whole food creations, especially my treats!

My Interests

When I look hard and find some free time, I enjoy learning, connecting with like-minded souls, spending time in and observing nature, walking, biking, practicing yoga, basking in the sunshine, swimming in warm, open water and dancing wildly, much to the dismay of my kids, especially if they have friends over☺. I love what I do. I meet the most amazing humans and I get to walk with my clients through their own life challenges and watch transformation happen before my eyes on a regular basis!!

If you were a fly on my wall, you'd notice how much I enjoy silence. You might find me attempting to garden, but getting lost in the joy of sinking my feet into the warm dirt and just sitting in it…bliss. You might catch me in my kitchen, otherwise known as my laboratory, making tantalizing and healthy food creations and offering them to those who have much experience with tasteless health food. I get a thrill from the positive reactions! You may also spy me spending time reading to my kids, teaching them to prepare healthy food or laughing at their mostly funny jokes. You would spend a lot of time watching me research and write, teaching classes and coaching clients back to a balanced life. Family, friends, good food, sunshine and my Creator are the things I hold most dear.

I am a certified Holistic Coach, Heart-Centered Hypnotherapist and CHEK Institute Holistic Lifestyle Coach. I offer retreats for transforming your relationship with food and healing those unhealed wounds that may cause self-sabotage in your life. You can find all of my services, recipes and blog at **www.mariarippo.com**.

As a young girl aspiring to share the good news of natural health, I dreamed of owning an island where the sun shines brightly and people from all walks of life could come to be rejuvenated. In a sense, The Green Smoothie Challenge is that island accessible to all who would like to come for a visit.

Welcome!

I'm so glad you came. It is my true hope that The Green Smoothie Challenge becomes a great blessing in your life. May you encounter abundant energy, improved health and joy in your accomplishment.

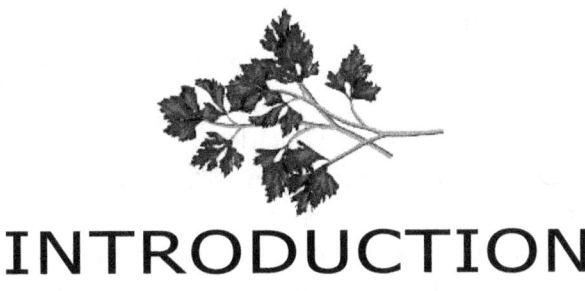

INTRODUCTION
What is The Green Smoothie Challenge?

The Green Smoothie Challenge is a body cleanse for busy people who have tried diet after diet only to become discouraged. It is a fresh way for you to increase your energy levels, clear your mind, release weight and improve your health. It is simple and affordable. And an experience that could change your life!

There are many motivations for desiring to accept a challenge such as this one. Upon reading the testimonials that follow, you will find that often people experience increased energy levels, significant weight-loss, improved ability to focus, silky smooth complexion, minimized food cravings, relief from back pain and the clearing up of unwanted symptoms of illness.

I developed The Original Green Smoothie Challenge to be a fast way for people to have a truly health-transforming experience. Simply put, it involves feasting only on green smoothies and munching on fresh fruit and veggie sticks, or steamed vegetables and vegetable soups for a designated time-period—one day, three days, five days or ten days. You are free to choose how long you would like to cleanse. Although I promote a few worldwide group Challenges on my website, you can take the Challenge as frequently or infrequently as you wish. Take it anytime that works for your personal schedule. Grab a group of friends to do it with or do it by yourself. It's completely up to you. Come to my Facebook page, **www.facebook.com/mariarippo**, to join a live Challenge throughout the year. Make sure to get 'notifications' so you can see when I start a Challenge! You are also invited to join my Facebook Group, The Green Smoothie Challenge at https://www.facebook.com/groups/1563334797230945/.

For some, this is a big step to take all at once. Because of this, I have developed a few ways to drastically improve your health and release weight easily and efficiently, while still being able to eat food along with drinking green smoothies. You will learn more about these options in Chapter 4. For now, I will discuss my Original Green Smoothie Challenge so you can decide if this sounds like a fit for you or if you'd rather start with a different option.

During the first option, the **Original Challenge**, you will be drinking up to seventy ounces of green smoothies per day. You may munch freely on celery, carrots, apples, jicama, cucumbers, bell peppers and other crunchy veggies that are appealing to you throughout the day. You may also eat an avocado or add it to your smoothie (I do this with flax or chia seeds and it holds me much longer). You will find all the smoothie recipes you need in the "Recipe" section of this guide. There you will find the exact smoothie recipes that allowed my husband and countless others to release fifteen pounds in nine days. You may follow these or make up your own. Also included are recipes from the Boutenko family, as well as a few others. You will simply prepare your entire day's worth of green smoothie in the morning and pack it up to take with you. Drink one-fourth of it at a time or divide it into smaller amounts to enjoy more often throughout the day.

Another great addition to your day during The Challenge is one or two freshly pressed juices. You will find recipes for these in Chapter 7 after the green smoothie recipes. Making fresh green juices does require a good juicer. I recommend the **Omega® juicer** or the **Champion®** (which is what I use). Using a good juicer is important, as it will keep the enzymes intact while the juice is extracted from the vegetables. If you do not own a juicer, feel free to skip this step. You are free to eat steamed or roasted vegetables as well as vegetable soup, especially if you are taking the Challenge during a colder season of the year.

The recipe section of Chapter 7 also includes my strawberry ice cream and chocolate milkshake recipes. You may enjoy one of these treats daily or every few days. Although they do not contain greens, they are very nutritious and will be a welcome addition to your Challenge! If you are sensitive to caffeine, it would be wise to skip the chocolate shake, as cocoa is a stimulant. Along with these treats, you are free to drink herbal teas and mineral water. You will also find my favorite mineral water 'cocktail' recipe along with the others mentioned above.

A very healing beverage is coconut kefir. **You can learn how to make it at www.youtube.com/GreenSmoothieCleanse**.

It's really that simple! Just mix, grab and go. Make sure you pack your fresh fruit and veggies to munch on when you get hungry.

If this Challenge seems too big of a step to take, no worries, you may customize your experience with three alternative Challenge options found in Chapter 4.

You can take The Green Smoothie Challenge anytime — one day a week, ten days a month or at the beginning of each year. You might also take it every other day or every third day intermittently, eating your normal diet on the days in between. Do it your way!

This book is written to be your guide and to give you recipes, encouragement, tools and more. Design your Challenge in a way that best fits your lifestyle and preferences. Do what *will* work for you as opposed to forcing yourself into taking too big of a step!

This is an amazing way to transform your health in a short, period of time. It is my hope that this Challenge, whichever version you choose to embark on, will not only help you to release weight, but also to gain a healthy relationship with the food you eat, to begin to feel which foods energize you and which suck the vitality out of you. I hope that by getting all the junk out of your amazingly beautiful and intelligent body for ten short days that you will see areas where you may be using food to numb your emotions instead of dealing with them in a healthy way. It is my hope that in ten short days you will feel clean, energized and excited about embarking on a new journey with food: healthy, life-giving, slimming and energizing food. It is my hope that you will begin to appreciate those foods that bring vitality and learn to recognize how food makes you feel so that you will never need to count a calorie again, but instead, simply eat the foods that make you look and feel great and honor your body by eating according to your hunger, i.e., eat only when you are good and hungry, and stop when you are just satisfied.

> *There are no incurable diseases. If you are willing to take responsibility for yourself and your life, you can heal yourself of anything. – Dr. Richard Schulze*

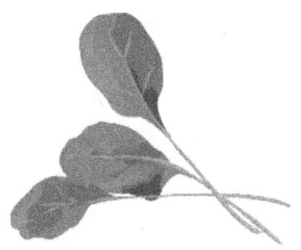

TESTIMONIALS

My initial involvement with green smoothies began a few years ago. I began to follow the story of a man named Clent Manich. Clent weighed about 400 pounds and had been given only a few years to live. He had type II diabetes. He had tried many diets, including a raw-food vegan diet. Even if he was successful at losing the weight, he would end up gaining it back and more. We'll begin the testimonial portion with a word from Dr. Donato, who inspired my involvement with green smoothies. Together with Victoria Boutenko, he helped Clent Manich lose over 200 lbs. in less than one year on green smoothies alone. Clent also lost all symptoms of diabetes while gaining back his health!

Dolphin's Raw Vegan Food Lifestyle Program as Explained by Dr. Miven Donato

Dolphin Health & Education is a clinical health and wellness center in Medford, Oregon. In my practice as a chiropractor and physical therapist, I see primarily orthopedic musculoskeletal conditions or disorders such as back pain, arthritis, work and sports injuries. Since the practice is also a wellness center, I see all kinds of chronic degenerative diseases such as obesity, cancer, diabetes (types I and II), osteoporosis, fibromyalgia, heart disease, lupus, pancreatic disease, thyroid problems, intestinal inflammations, colitis, IBS, chronic fatigue syndrome, immune deficiency problems, allergy problems and anything to do with low energy conditions. I also see fairly healthy people who want to learn how to maximize health and longevity.

Clent Manich was a client referred to me by a physician. He had injured his low back. I routinely see low back pain cases but Clent was a special case in that he was grossly obese. At 396 pounds there was not a whole lot I could do for him in terms of spinal adjustments. I showed him a few stretches and strengthening exercises for his back. But the bottom line was his weight. Ultimately if he could lose a significant amount of weight, most of his back pain would be resolved. I was more interested in his overall health, while he was only interested in getting rid of the pain. So when I discussed my plans for him, he thought about it and was agreeable to follow Dolphin's Raw-Food, Vegan Lifestyle Program as a long-term approach to solving the back pain but also losing weight quickly and getting his health back.

Going raw is NEVER easy! At Dolphin, I start people at 85% raw and 15% cooked in terms of the food that is consumed within a 24-hour period. Clent went into the 10-week intensive raw-vegan food lifestyle program, which is now known as Dolphin's Healthy Boot Camp. He started at 85% raw. At the end of the boot camp, he'd lost 52 pounds. However, he was not able to keep up the raw-food lifestyle over time and eventually lost his direction. The second time around, a year later, he went all raw focusing on the green smoothies, vegetables and fruits. This time he was more successful. He lost 225 pounds within 1 year. He gained more than his health back. It gave him confidence and motivation in life. He started all raw at 401 pounds and went down to his lowest at 176 pounds in exactly one year. I monitored him consistently about once a week. I also coached him through the exercise program. I learned a lot from that entire experience. The program was very successful in his situation. I am constantly upgrading and/or revising the lifestyle program to make it easier and safer to follow.

There are dangers associated from losing too much weight in a short period. The individuals more at risk are usually the ones taking medications for high blood pressure, diabetes, heart disease, etc. The more medications (prescription or over-the-counter) taken while in the raw vegan lifestyle, the more potential for problems to occur. Dizziness or blacking out can occur. Individuals on Coumadin must first consult with their physicians before going on green smoothies or green drinks. Gall bladder inflammation or gall stone attacks can occur and will have to be dealt with appropriately. Individuals following a high raw-vegan food diet must be responsible and knowledgeable or should be properly monitored especially within *the first six to eight months for any disabling symptoms or complications due to detoxification.*

Rapid weight loss occurs when people follow a high-raw plant-based diet because the caloric intake and fat intake are generally reduced. Rapid weight-loss is safe as long as the nutrient density in the diet is high, there is no interference in transport and cellular uptake and the body is getting the necessary nourishment. The Standard American Diet (SAD) does not supply the body with the high nutrient density food that is found in the high raw plant-based diet and can therefore lead to malnutrition, chemical imbalances, and diseases of nutrient deficiency and/or chemical toxicity besides the rapid weight loss when food portions are reduced. On the other hand, responsible people who follow a high-raw, plant-based diet are eating bulkier unaltered, uncooked fiber foods that are lower in caloric density, attain a normal weight. The factors that need to be considered when losing weight in the raw vegan lifestyle in terms of food, are adequate quantity, high quality and variety. Combined with a good exercise program and proper hydration.

Dr. Miven Donato

Doctor of Physical Therapy

Doctor of Chiropractic

Although many people have successfully released weight and gained their health back through a raw-vegan diet, I do not recommend this for long term. I have seen it work well for one year, especially when one is so addicted to food that they just need a complete break from the availability of the foods they are addicted to, as in the case of Clent, who needed to go off of all food for a sufficient enough time that he no longer desired to eat the foods that were literally killing him. I highly recommend being under the care of a qualified practitioner when making drastic changes to one's diet.

Following are some letters I've received from people who have benefitted greatly from taking The Green Smoothie Challenge:

My name is Lisa. I never had a weight problem until after my second child was born. Before then, I could eat pretty much what I liked and as long as I would exercise, I had no weight issue. But, after my son was born, when I was thirty-seven, I just couldn't lose any weight, no matter what I tried. I felt awful, tired, was puffy all the time and even began to feel depressed. After trying many of the boxed meal diet systems, fasting, low-carb diets and everything in between, I had just about given up on myself. I felt awful. But then my sister, Maria Rippo, told me about a man named Clent who worked for Costco and had been grossly obese. He had a myriad of health problems. He went on a green smoothie diet and lost over 200 pounds. All of his health issues disappeared. I looked at his website and read everything I could. I thought it sounded like something I could do.

At first, I tried having a green smoothie for breakfast, and then another for lunch and eating a snack and then dinner. I didn't lose any weight, or really feel any different at first. So, my sister suggested that I try 100% green smoothies. I did it and lost 9 pounds in 13 days. I did have a handful of almonds twice a day besides the green smoothies. Then, after 3 weeks, I went to a green smoothie for breakfast, a raw salad for lunch and either a green smoothie for dinner or a piece of grilled fish or chicken with vegetables. I lost 22 pounds in about 8 weeks and feel great. My husband and friends say my skin just glows, I am no longer puffy, I have lots of energy, and the best part is, after the first two weeks, I lost my craving for refined carbohydrates and sugar! Those were my junk foods of choice, and I do just fine without them now!

I just have to say that I've become addicted to green smoothies. I've been doing them almost all week and losing about a pound a day, so wonderful. I wish I'd discovered them sooner... I lost a lot of weight. Stress, coffee and sugar do not mix well with my body! I was an instant fan of the green smoothies! I wanted to cleanse my body and lose some excess pounds in the process. It was so easy, just open the fridge, grab the veggies & fruit, blend and add some flax or hemp. I'm super busy and having all three meals in one container I can drink on the go was awesome! The best part for me was that I lost more than a pound a day! I haven't lost it that fast in years! – Elizabeth R.

Whenever I feel as if I need to get back on track, I go on the green smoothies for 3-5 days and I feel so clean and light. I have 10 more pounds to lose, and I know I will be there soon. I highly encourage anyone to try The Green Smoothie Challenge and see just how light and clean you feel! – Lisa O.

Doing a green smoothie cleanse was a great experience and really it was surprisingly simple. It was also really nice to have Maria as a support person. She was very knowledgeable and quick to answer any questions that I had. Furthermore, Maria was such an encourager. I chose to do a 3-day green smoothie cleanse, but ended up feeling so good I went one extra day.

The use of kale and spinach were my vegetable base every day and each day I varied the fruit I put in my smoothie. I tried to make it 40% vegetable and 60% fruit. I used my high-speed blender to make my smoothies, which crushed the ice really nicely. I often made my biggest smoothie in the morning and then put what I couldn't eat in the refrigerator until later in the day. The smoothies actually kept well in the refrigerator, which surprised me. I am one of those people who likes to have a crunch added to my eating experience, so at times I felt a bit tempted, but I would snack on carrots or broccoli to help add that crunch. I also occasionally had half of an avocado with a little bit of seasoning on it to help curb my hunger.

I really am amazed at the benefits of this in such a short time. I lost 7 pounds in 4 days! I am now at the weight I was when I was in high school! Even more than that, I had an amazing amount of energy and just felt better. Taking everything out of my diet except these greens and fruit took away the temptation to run to the cookie jar for something sweet—my body needed a little break from that. Anyway since I have completed my smoothie cleanse, I am actually craving green smoothies. During my 4 days, I continued to work out like I normally do. I noticed that each day further into the cleanse I had more energy than the day before and was able to soar through workouts with tons of energy and was able to keep my heart rate up higher than normal.

I plan to make having a green smoothie part of my regular daily routine! Thanks Maria for all of your inspiration! – Cheryl M.

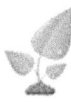

Last February I noticed a friend looking very good and asked her what she had been doing. She told me about the green smoothies and Maria. That same day I went home and read about it. Besides losing weight, the cleanse had helped others with problems like complexion, feeling bloated, lethargic and many other ailments that I was facing as well. So I bought Maria's book and started that same day. I did the 10-day challenge and found it so refreshing. I was able to stick with it better than anything else I've ever tried. I thought I was a healthy eater before, but realized my body was missing out on all the benefits of raw fruits, vegetables and nuts. I had so much energy, lost 10 pounds and my complexion improved. But there was something unexpected that came from it as well. I had been trying to get pregnant for eight months and about the time I started the challenge I figured it wasn't going to happen, but just a couple weeks after doing the challenge, I was PREGNANT! I know it was all due to the green smoothie cleanse. I now have at least one smoothie a day and eat more raw fruits and veggies, along with my kids who are often picky eaters! I truly feel this has changed my life and now have hope that I can get my pregnancy weight off as well as feel great and have a healthy family. Thanks so much Maria, you are an inspiration! – Kelly J

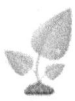

I began The Green Smoothie Challenge because I felt tired, overweight and wanted to get back in shape. I wasn't happy about where I was mentally or physically, so I decided to jump in one day and take the 10-day Challenge—after all, what's ten days if I'm really going to change the way I look and feel! The first four days were the most difficult. I really wanted to eat and was frustrated with myself for having committed to doing it. But I knew I had to stick with it and really see for myself if this was going to work. Dinnertime was the hardest time of day for me as I strongly craved all the food that we were preparing for the family. This was definitely the toughest part, much more so than I originally thought. I really had to mentally work through the mind games surrounding the desire to give in. I stuck with it, and I was glad I did. I began to lose weight immediately, three pounds the first day!

The results on the scale each day kept me going and helped me to stick with it and not give in to my longing to eat. I was amazed, but it's really true: there is a way to get healthier and lose weight all at once, and it is The Green Smoothie Challenge. I began to feel a lot more energy by about day five. I started wanting to get outside and run or hit the gym. I've never been one to go to the gym, and I found myself really craving a good workout. My mind became sharper, I lost that daily three o'clock slump, and did not need as much sleep as normal. My wife says I stopped snoring completely. All of these things began to outweigh any craving I had to eat food. I lost fifteen pounds in nine days and have continued to lose more weight as I still drink a lot of green smoothies during the week.

Once I accomplished the challenge, I created my own personal plan of incorporating green smoothies into my diet. I continue to get great results and feel amazing. I've settled in on a weekly plan to keep me on track, which is to enjoy myself reasonably on the weekends and balance it during the week with a healthy dose of green smoothies. Specifically, I do a three-day challenge each week on Tuesday, Wednesday and Thursday. On Friday, I drink green smoothies and then enjoy eating dinner. Saturday and Sunday I eat sensibly, and Monday, I drink green smoothies and eat a light dinner.

This cycle is now working for my schedule and allows for fun, light wining and dining on the weekends. The great thing about The Challenge is once you do it, it grows on you and you crave healthier foods for your body. I am now down twenty pounds and feel great. I highly recommend taking The Green Smoothie Challenge for ten days; you'll see and experience what I'm talking about – Tobin R

The morning after Day 1 of my 15 day Green Smoothie Challenge, my eyes almost popped out of my head when I hopped on the scale. Five pounds in one day! I hadn't been able to lose weight for years! Day one had been challenging, but after seeing results like that, I was excited to keep going. I started The Challenge to see if I could get rid of my candida symptoms, reduce the puffiness in my face and see if I actually could lose a few pounds. (Ok, more than just a few!) Days 2 and 3 proved tough, though, because I missed getting to feel satisfied by hearty meals, felt weak and exhausted, and I didn't see any more progress on the scale. Maria encouraged me to keep on going, and was quite the faithful cheerleader! So I stuck with it, and pretty soon things evened out, and I began losing about a pound each day.

Then Thanksgiving came, and along with it, the emotional roller coaster of frustration from not getting to join the family feast! I knew The Challenge was good for me, and I had committed to sticking to it, but that was ridiculously tough. Watching my family soak up homemade syrup the next morning with Grandpa's famous waffles was the worst of the worst, and seemed like the climax of The Challenge.

After I successfully said "no" to that, I was more confident in my ability to "keep on trucking!" and looked forward to what sort of new combination of fruits and greens I could come up with. My candida and psoriasis symptoms completely disappeared as the days progressed, the energy started kicking in and when my roommates returned from their Thanksgiving travels and completely freaked out when they saw the change in my figure, I decided the whole adventure was worth it. It was now a race to see how many more days I could push through. My first goal was 10, but then I decided to try for 15. My roommates joined me, and we all started feeling so much healthier, craving the dark leafy greens and bouncing off the walls with excitement for how well our clothes were fitting!

While the hard part was still having to say "no" to Christmas party treats, and getting a little tired of avocados and tomatoes, I continually was re-encouraged by the fast and always-exciting loss of weight, and by friends and students who would ask, "Is there something different about you? You look different!"

After 15 days, having lost a total of 14 pounds, I let myself enjoy the food I so badly missed. But after two days of eating "normally," I definitely saw the difference. My energy disappeared, my face started getting puffy again and I just didn't feel as excited about the day ahead. So, I've pulled the blender back out, stocked up on Swiss Chard, mangoes, avocados, pears, spinach, and some frozen blackberries, and here I am, sipping away on a kind of purple-colored Green Smoothie! And I'm thrilled. The Green Smoothie Challenge is life changing and has caused me to want to change the way I eat for good! – Rachel R.

After being on two Green Smoothie Challenges since the beginning of last April, I've lost more than 15 lbs., made it through the holidays without gaining more than a few pounds and have gotten off of a statin drug! Now that's something to celebrate! I think they're grrrreat! – Martha W.

I have been researching green smoothies for a while now. I have learned a lot and wanted to make a big change in my diet. I am getting married in less than 2 months and wanted to get in better shape and learn about healthier foods to make for my future family. Somehow I convinced my fiancé to join me in a healthier way of living. We started drinking two green smoothies a day; it has been 19 days now. We both have more energy; we don't get tired during the day; we're happier and healthier. We have both lost about five pounds already and haven't gotten sick at all. I've never felt this great before!! Right before I started this green smoothie diet/challenge I got a UTI and didn't go to the doctor…after three days of green smoothies my UTI was gone without seeing a doctor or taking any medication!!! I told my co-workers in Blendtec™ Customer Service about my experience with this new lifestyle/diet and so far two of my co-workers have started the challenge as well – Emily Call

I will be 44 years old in a couple of months. Last year in November, I came back from a holiday and anxiously weighed myself. (I hadn't weighted myself in months.) Eeeck, I had gained 15 pounds in about one and a half years. It was the most I had weighed in my entire life. It was time to really do something.

I had noticed since I hit my 40s that it had become more difficult to maintain my weight. It was a struggle to lose just five pounds, where as before I could lose it easily in a week or so. I am one of those people who could always eat just about anything I wanted, and if I gained a little, I would lose it easily. I was exercising pretty regularly by running on the treadmill a couple days a week and going to yoga a few days a week, but nothing major. I am a pretty active person i.e.: dog walks, long walks with my husband, and gardening. So, I started scouring the Internet to see what was out there, and I came upon The Green Smoothie Challenge. I bought the e-book and after reading it knew I had to try this cleanse/diet. It seemed so easy and healthy.

Maria makes it so easy by giving you a shopping list of ingredients to buy. I ran out to the market immediately and bought everything I needed for the first five days of the challenge. I started the challenge the next morning.

It was amazing; I lost two pounds the first day and continued to lose weight every single day. In all, I lost around 10 pounds and three and a half inches around my waist.

Not only did I lose weight but I felt so good. No indigestion, bloating or even major hunger pains. I also had more energy. I drank the smoothies and ate cut-up fresh fruit and veggies in between. I did have a headache the second day, probably because of caffeine or sugar withdrawal. Dinnertime was kind of tough, but I powered through it because I was seeing such great results. Seeing my weight drop every morning was great incentive.

I had tried a couple other cleanses in the past and didn't like them. With the other cleanses I was constantly running to the bathroom. It was horrible and the stuff they wanted you to drink was disgusting.

The above is the first time I did the challenge. I decided to do it a second time and join in the Worldwide Green Smoothie Challenge, starting Jan. 3, 2011. We had over-indulged at Christmas and New Years. I had gained back 3 of the 10 pounds I lost and still wanted to lose a few extra on top of that. I had the same amazing results this second time. I lost eight pounds, and I am closer to my ideal weight of a couple years ago.

Something important I noticed this second time around was such clarity of mind that was really neat. This second time around I didn't have the cravings I had the first time, and I knew to watch what I ate and drank a few days before I started this challenge. No headache this time.

I continue to drink the smoothies during the day and eat a balanced meal at dinnertime. The Green Smoothies will be a permanent part of my life: so easy, so healthy, and a great way to maintain my weight. A number of my friends have tried it and love it; they just can't believe how well they feel and how easy it is.

I need to mention how supportive Maria is. She always replies to emails and Facebook posts with great information, tips and encouragement. Thank you so much Maria. As far as I am concerned, these smoothies are a miracle. I just wish I had found you sooner. – Katheryn Leszczynski

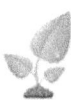

My name is Japhy and I went on Maria's program, 'The Green Smoothie Challenge' right after Christmas 2012 from December 26th to January 4th. Before beginning 'The Challenge', I weighed in at 243 pounds and my fasting Blood Sugar was at 204. I have Type-2 Diabetes and so I need to monitor my blood sugars daily. Before beginning one of Maria's programs called 'The Green Smoothie Challenge', I loved my sweets like candy bars, cookies and cakes. During 'The Challenge', I was drinking 3-4 quarts of Green Smoothie per day. In addition to the smoothies, I would have the occasional apple and perhaps some celery and cucumbers at night with Guacamole. The big difference was...there was NO SUGAR as in candy bars, cookies etc. during my 10-day 'Challenge.' The great new is that by day 5 of 'The Challenge', I was OFF my Metformin Diabetes meds and I was dropping weight every day. At the end of the 10 -day challenge, I had lost 10 pounds and had normalized my blood sugar to a reading of '101.' In short...taking the sugar out of my diet and adding green smoothies was highly successful and I continue on that course today a month later after ending the challenge. I worked with Maria daily during my ten day Challenge and continue to work with her daily via email and weekly phone appointments. The greatest part is that I can tell the work I am doing is permanent. At my one-month mark of doing this work, I am down to 219 lbs. and have now gone off of my blood pressure meds as well. I no longer crave the foods that were keeping me overweight and craving foods that were quite literally killing me. I highly recommend working with Maria. – Japhy Whalen

HERE WE GO!

Congratulations! You are about to begin a journey that may take you places you have yet to travel. Oftentimes it is our challenges that strengthen us more than anything else can. The Green Smoothie Challenge may test your personal limits. It is simple but may *not* be easy.

This may be the biggest challenge you have ever taken on. As you persevere down this path, you may experience trials. Overcoming these trials has the ability to reveal some strengths you possess that you may not have been aware of until now. These strengths may not begin to reveal themselves until after four, five, or even six days on the Challenge. At first the road may seem mostly uphill, a very steep hill, for some. One thing I know is that you *can* do this. You *will* be amazed at the results. As long as you know beforehand that it will be very challenging at times, you will persevere. And when completed, you'll experience a victory unlike any you've experienced before. I highly recommend doing this Challenge along with your family, a friend or a group of friends.

Days one, two and three may be the most challenging part of your experience. It is a time of readjustment for your body, which has been accustomed to receiving calories externally from food. Now it must shift to receiving small amounts of highly nutritious food and using up its stored resources for energy. Allow your body to get through this period. It may beg you for food (in a very earnest manner!), which can cause discomfort. Many of us are not accustomed to enduring the feeling of hunger. It can cause panic. As Tom Venuto, author of *Burn the Fat, Feed the Muscle,* likes to say: "Hunger is not an emergency." Allow these first few days to pass. Slowly but surely, as your body grows accustomed to new energy sources (namely, consuming it's own fat for energy!) and your stomach contracts, it will stop asking for so much food and will be quite content with the amazing, life-giving nutrients its receiving and your mind may feel more clear than it ever has. In these first few days, your body is actually going through withdrawal from foods you may be addicted or allergic to.

Because you are only eating blended foods and raw fruits along with raw or steamed vegetables, you are giving your digestive system a considerable break. When you give this gift to your body, you free it up to do "repair" work. Your body will go to work cleansing and healing. One reason it can do this is that green smoothies are very rich in **enzymes**. According to Ann Wigmore, natural health pioneer and founder of the world renowned Hippocrates Health Institute, "… if it is weight-loss you are after, or reversal of any other form of deposit in the body such as calcium in arthritis, excess protein in tumors, or cholesterol in atherosclerosis, only enzymes do the work of breaking them up and eliminating them." I will go into more detail about enzymes a little later.

Albert Einstein said, "The definition of insanity is doing the same thing over and over again and expecting different results." If you desire to become more healthy and energetic or to weigh less than you do, then you must do something differently than you are currently doing. So why not give The Green Smoothie Challenge a try and see what kinds of amazing results you can get?

[2] Wigmore, Ann, *The Hippocrates Diet and Health Program*. Avery Publishing Group Inc., Wayne, NJ. 1984.

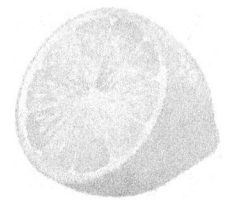

CHAPTER 1
Meet the Green Smoothie

What is a Green Smoothie?

The green smoothie is a delicious and refreshing beverage invented by Victoria Boutenko, raw-food pioneer, chef, author and educator. Boutenko's family suffered greatly with different diseases, and both she and her husband were given very short, periods of time to live. One of their children, Sergei, had diabetes and the doctor advised him to begin taking insulin. Another child suffered from asthma. At her wits end and not wanting her husband to endure one more surgery, Victoria turned to raw, living foods and almost immediately improved the health of her family. Healed of the diseases that once plagued them, this family now lives vibrantly healthy lives.

At one point, the Boutenkos realized they didn't eat enough greens. Eating more nutrition-packed greens became their goal but eating so many seemed a chore. Boutenko decided to try "hiding" them in a smoothie. When they began consuming a quart daily, they noticed even more health improvements. Because making the green smoothie is so simple and enormously health enhancing, it has become a very popular addition to any healthy diet.

A green smoothie, in simple terms, is a delicious fruit smoothie with dark, leafy greens or other vegetables added to it. A good place to start is with a smoothie made from 40% vegetables and 60% fruit. Any leafy-green and fruit combination is acceptable. I will also teach you about other healthy vegetables you might like to add. As you get used to drinking this delightful beverage, you may choose to work towards adding 60% vegetables and 40% fruit or even less.

Here is a sample green smoothie recipe:

1 banana   3 handfuls spinach   2 cups strawberries

3 leaves kale   1 apple

Simply add all of the above ingredients to your blender (you may need to do it in two batches), and then fill the blender about half way with pure, filtered or spring water and blend. Enjoy.

> **Caution:** Taking in too much of one kind of greens for an extended time period can have a toxic effect because greens contain a small amount of alkaloids. The good news is that different greens contain different alkaloids so as long as you switch them up each day you'll have no problem with this. You can even switch them up each week. For example, you can have spinach one day, romaine the next, kale the next, etc., or you can have spinach one week, kale the next, romaine the next, and so on. I even make smoothies with no greens and instead I substitute cucumbers, celery and zucchini and maybe some parsley or cilantro. There is not a right or wrong to do this, so make sure you find the best way for YOU!

Why Green Smoothies?

It is commonly accepted as safe and health promoting for a person to live on fruits and vegetables alone for a short, period of time. Taking The Green Smoothie Challenge shows, more than anything else I have seen, the energizing and health-enhancing effect that eating a diet rich in enzyme-rich, fresh, living foods as well as, or possibly more importantly, removing all the damaging foods from one's diet, can have on a person's health. There truly is no other way to experience this so quickly. It is my hope for you to feel and see the powerful difference made by consuming only living foods, for a short period of time. I have often heard it said that it's not so much what you *do* eat that makes you healthy, it's what you *don't* eat that's important. Taking the Challenge allows for an opportunity to take all the junk out of your system for 10 straight days and the results can tend to be quite miraculous. It is a very fast way to experience the energy and vitality you can feel, when less-than-optimal foods are removed from your diet.

Hippocrates, the father of modern-day medicine said, "Let thy food by thy medicine and thy medicine be thy food." I have seen this simple piece of profound advice become true before my eyes many, many times. I watch people's health transform when they remove processed carbohydrates, refined sugars, pasteurized dairy products, table salt and refined vegetable oils from their diets and replace them with a large amount of green, enzyme-rich foods among other healthy foods.

I am often amazed at the careful attention people pay to their cars, putting in the best oil, quality gasoline, getting lube jobs regularly, and the like. Our bodies are immensely more complicated than our cars. However, some choose to ignore the statistics and put damaging foods into their systems on a regular basis. This is not right or wrong, but it is important to understand the positive and negative consequences of such decisions and make mindful choices about how we treat our amazing bodies. The Green Smoothie Challenge makes it simple to take a break from these less-than-optimal foods and experience how our body feels with a fresh, clean start in a short, period of time. The 10-day Challenge is ideal for feeling the true benefits. Once you have made it five days, getting to ten is easy because you have already made it through the most challenging part. After five days, you may only have experienced the immense challenges of going off of what may be very addicting foods. It is only *after* five or six days that you may begin to notice dramatic changes. This is very similar to having surgery, where often, the pain on the third and fourth day is more intense than on the first or second day. Often, we feel worse before we feel better, much like having withdrawals from any addictive substance. One may face more pain before feeling better.

The health benefits of green smoothies are tremendous. The American Cancer Society recommends that we "eat five or more servings of a variety of vegetables and fruits each day." The green smoothie makes this goal attainable. It literally takes less than ten minutes to make and clean up. It is very affordable at a cost of about $8.00 – $12.00 per day for the organic version while on the Challenge.

The main reason green smoothies are so healthy is, well, they are green! And green, for lack of a better word, is good!

Leafy green vegetables are some of the most nutrient dense foods we can put into our bodies. The amount of greens you consume is associated with successful, long-term weight control and good health. The more you eat, the better your rate of success! Because of their bulk, they also help us feel full and therefore, eat less! The question I am asked most often about taking The Green Smoothie Challenge is: "Where will I get my protein?" Have you ever wondered where cows, gorillas and horses get their protein? Of course, we are not cows, gorillas or horses, but these are big animals with large muscles. They need their protein too. (And no, I am not suggesting you go out to your lawn to get your greens!) Greens happen to be very high in **protein**, as well as rich in other important nutrients such as **fiber**, **chlorophyll** and the number one health restorer of them all—**enzymes**. Green smoothies are also incredibly **hydrating** as well as being full of **vitamins** and **minerals**. This is a main reason why so many people notice a

---

[3]http://www.cancer.org/docroot/PED/content/PED_3_2X_Diet_and_Activity_Factors_That_Affect_Risks.asp

[4] Furhman, Dr. Joel, MD, Eat to Live: The Revolutionary Formula for Fast and Sustained Weight Loss, Little, Brown and Company. Hatchet Book Group, Park Avenue, New York, NY. 2003.

transformation in their skin. Often, people become hydrated for the first time. They are also adding a large amount of **alkaline forming foods** to their diet in the form of dark leafy greens. In addition, Greens are full of **anti-cancer nutrients**. All of these factors contribute to good health and longevity. Another important property of leafy greens is their high amount of **biophotons**, which are stored light energy from the sun.

Dark leafy green vegetables are made of about half protein! Each leafy green vegetable has certain amino acids, but when our diet consists of a good variety of leafy greens, we end up getting a wide variety of amino acids to enable our bodies to properly build proteins. I believe we also need quality animal protein in order to thrive, but for a temporary, period of time, it can be very beneficial to take a break from it. Because greens are highly nutrient dense and because they have so much fiber, they are considered an effective addition to any weight-loss plan. The high fiber and chlorophyll content also makes them an important choice for cleansing our bodies. This is not to say that green smoothies should be considered our only protein source, but they are a good source of plant protein.

Let's examine each of these important elements more closely.

Fiber is a very important ingredient in any healthy diet. It is vital not so much because of the nutritional value that it offers, but for its cleansing effect. Fiber acts as a "sweeper truck," cleaning debris from the colon walls. It moves through our colon absorbing waste and clearing it away—eliminating it on its way out. Greens can absorb up to three times their weight in toxins that are then removed from the body. A buildup of toxins in the body causes unwanted side effects such as acne, sickness, disease and weight gain. Keeping the colon running properly through an adequate intake of fiber is one of the most important things you can do for your health. People who add green smoothies to their diet tell me they have never had such an amazing ability to eliminate. The other notable difference is in the skin. The first thing you will notice, when you look at someone who has been on The Challenge, is their beautiful skin. Now, that's a beauty secret we don't hear enough about! The enzymes keep you young as well. Where else can you get all of this for eight bucks a day?

According to the Oxford English Dictionary, **chlorophyll** is "the colouring matter of the leaves and other green parts of plants; found in the cells usually in the form of minute granules (*chlorophyll-bodies* or *-corpuscles*)." I've found using a high-power blender is the best way to make the green smoothie because it is powerful enough to break the cell walls of the leafy greens so the chlorophyll is readily available for the body to absorb. Chlorophyll purifies the blood. It most closely represents the hemoglobin in human blood, making it very similar to our own blood. Your body uses chlorophyll for

---

[5] http://dictionary.oed.com 2nd Edition 1989, Oxford University Press.

cleansing and healing its organs, battling pathogenic bacteria, and supplying oxygen wherever it is needed. Chlorophyll is a strong immune system strengthener. The greener a leaf is, the more chlorophyll it contains. Now you know why your mom always told you to eat your spinach. There really is a reason! The good news is that green smoothies taste much more delightful than cooked spinach. The secret of the green smoothie is you "sneak" many greens into a fruit smoothie and taste only the flavors of the fruit. Shhh, your taste buds will never know!

Proteins are the building blocks of life. If proteins are the building blocks, amino acids are the grains of sand and clay from which the blocks are made. According to Norman Walker, DSc, "Fruits and vegetables contain the necessary atoms from which amino acids are formed in the system." These atoms, when ingested from fresh produce, are what the body uses to actually manufacture amino acids and proteins. There is a big difference between eating raw foods and fully cooked foods. The cooked foods require a 'breaking down' process in the body because the enzymes in the food are cooked out. This is very important to understand because this "breaking down" process also involves manufacturing and using up enzyme stores in your body. This is the main cause of aging. Once you have done this Challenge for ten days, you will notice amazing changes in your skin. This is partly because you are giving your body a much-needed break from the hard work of digesting cooked foods. Your improved skin will be the proof! Don't misunderstand here, I am not saying to stop eating cooked foods, but more that we must begin adding 'living' foods into our diets of cooked foods.

Enzymes are involved in every process of your being. Ann Wigmore, founder of the world renowned Hippocrates Health Institute says, "Every breath you take, thought you think, or sentence you read, is a result of thousands of complex enzyme systems and their functions operating simultaneously. They are active construction and demolition teams that work twenty-four hours a day to maintain health and balance in your body." Enzymes are the labor force of the body.They are vitally important to your state of health and yet, many people don't know anything about their significance. Enzymes are found in raw, living foods including both plant and animal sources (living foods are those that remain in their natural, raw state and have not been heated above 118° F). Some examples are **lacto-fermented sauerkraut**, sashimi, raw milk kefir and yogurts, sprouts, raw fruits and veggies, raw nuts and seeds, etc. Enzymes are destroyed at

---

[6] Boutenko, Victoria, Green for Life. Ashland, OR; Raw Family Publishing, 2005

[7] "amino acid." Britannica Student Encyclopedia. Encyclopedia Britannica Online Library Edition. Encyclopedia Britannica, 2009. Web. 8 Dec. 2009 <http://library.eb.com/kids/comptons/article-9272835>.

[8] Walker, N.W., D. Sc, The Vegetarian Guide to Diet and Salad, Prescott, AZ, Norwalk Press, 1971

[9] Ibid

[10] Wigmore, Ann, The Hippocrates Diet and Health Program, Avery Publishing Group Inc., Wayne, NJ. 1984.

[11] Ibid

temperatures above 118° Fahrenheit. They enable us to digest and assimilate our foods. If we consume cooked foods regularly, our bodies must manufacture their own enzymes in order to digest and break down our food. Eventually we begin to run low on our enzyme stores. This process causes aging and disease when it occurs on a regular basis. By giving our bodies living, enzyme-rich foods, we can be healthier and stay younger longer. Lack of enzymes in the diet contributes to a buildup of undigested food in the colon, which creates a breeding ground for infection, toxic bacteria and autointoxication.

In 1939, Francis N. Pottenger, Jr, MD, did a study with cats to see how well they would survive on a diet of cooked foods. By the third generation the cats fed on totally cooked cat chow as opposed to those fed raw animal foods, were so severely malnourished they were unable to reproduce. Because the cats were deficient in enzymes, they were unable to digest food and had become malnourished. To further illustrate this point, one only need look at the fact that the United States was formerly a nation of orphanages, but has now turned to a nation of fertility clinics. Could living on a mostly cooked, processed and genetically modified-food diet have something to do with the phenomenon? I think there is a direct correlation!

As I mentioned earlier, when we mix greens in a high-speed blender, the cell walls break down and the benefits of the greens are easily assimilated into our systems. The cell walls must be broken in order for the chlorophyll to become available. The digestion process begins in the mouth. It is important to drink the smoothie slowly and to actually chew it a little bit so it can mix with your saliva to initiate the digestive process before you even swallow! I personally use the **Blendtec™ blender** as it also breaks open the cell walls of the produce.

Hydration. According to Dr. Brian Clement of the Hippocrates Health Institute, "many of us aren't getting enough water." Shocking, but Clement says that it's estimated that 60 percent of the world's population doesn't drink enough water to keep the cells hydrated and the body healthy. Even more, as many as 40 percent of people lack the mechanism in the brain that tells them to drink when their bodies are really thirsty. Instead of waiting for your thirst signs, take hydration breaks throughout the day and keep a tall glass of H_2O at your desk." It is widely thought that drinking twice your body weight in ounces of water per day is necessary for proper hydration.

Hydration is one of the most overlooked keys to vibrant health. In order for normal

---

[12] Huntoon, Jenefer ND. (January 19, 2009). "Enzymes: The Missing Key to Health." Retrieved February 19, 2011 from: Plant Enzymes: A Key to Health web site: http://enzymesakey.blogspot.com/

[13] Jio, Sarah, (January 20, 2011). "5 Things I learned from the New Book, Crazy, Sexy Diet." Retrieved May 18, 2011 from the Glamour Health and Fitness Web site: http://www.glamour.com/health-fitness/blogs/vitamin-g/2011/01/5-things-i-learned-from-the-ne.html#ixzz1FfkC6hC0

physiological and digestive processes to occur, our bodies must be properly hydrated. Fruits and vegetables are some of the most hydrating foods we can eat. They contain perfectly structured water that is easily absorbed by the cells. Some common symptoms of dehydration include cravings for sugar, cravings for salt on your food, feeling dehydrated and thirsty with a need to drink plenty of water, difficulty falling asleep at night, sleeping lightly or waking early or often, difficulty relaxing, feeling nervous, anxious or hyperactive, constipation and general exhaustion. By nature, green smoothies are hydrating. Drinking green smoothies and eating plenty of raw foods in their natural form for ten days can be a great help in reversing symptoms of dehydration. According to author and holistic health practitioner, Paul Chek, dehydration affects the health of the stomach and intestines, interfering with digestion and often causing acid reflux. He says that heartburn is a sign of dehydration. This may be why so many people are relieved of their heartburn so quickly when they take The Challenge.

Vitamins and Minerals are essential for optimal health. They are plentiful in leafy green vegetables. Leafy greens contain every nutrient we need including all vitamins, minerals and amino acids except for vitamin B-12. It is important to note that although leafy greens have such an amazing nutritional make-up, our diets must consist of a large variety of foods in order to experience optimal health. Current research points to the fact that it is much more effective to get our vitamins and minerals from high quality, whole-food sources rather than from supplementation. It has also shown that we must eat certain animal fats in order to absorb the minerals. These foods include organ meats, butter, lard and cod-liver oil which contain the fat soluble vitamins A, D, E and K that are the carriers of minerals into our teeth, bones and body. When I was on a totally raw food diet, I became very mineral deficient because my diet lacked these all-important fats.

Anti-Cancer Nutrients. "In a review of 206 human-population studies, raw vegetable consumption showed the strongest protective effect against cancer of any beneficial food." Dark, leafy green vegetables are known to be high in antioxidants and phytochemicals, both powerful against cancer.

Alkalinity. Food either creates an acidic or an alkaline condition in the body. Leafy greens are very alkalinizing to the body. It is said that disease thrives in an acidic environment.

There are a few diets out there that claim to cure type I and II diabetes using the method

[14] http://www.bodyecology.com/07/04/19/dehydrated.php

[15] Chek, Paul, How to Eat, Move and Be Healthy, A Chek Institute Publication, San Diego, CA. 2004.

[16] Boutenko, Victoria, Green Smoothie Revolution, North Atlantic Books, Berkeley, CA 2009.

[17] Fuhrman, Dr. Joel, Eat to Live: The Revolutionary approach Formula for Fast and Sustained Weight Loss, Little, Brown and Company, New York, NY. 2003.

of alkalinizing the body. Alkaline diets have also been successful in the treatment of osteoporosis. Equally important in reversing diabetes is eating the proper fats, and plenty of them while eliminating all processed foods.

Biophotons are "small units of life stored by every organic organism, including you." "Stored sun energy finds its way into our cells via food in the form of minute particles of light. These light particles are called 'biophotons', which are the smallest physical units of light. According to Professor F.A. Popp, founder of the International Institute of Biophysics in Neuss, Germany and Dr. H. Niggli, a Swiss photobiologist, biophotons contain important bio-information, which controls complex vital processes in our bodies. The biophotons have the power to order and regulate, and, in doing so, to elevate the organism to a higher oscillation or order. This is manifested as a feeling of vitality and well-being." Leafy green vegetables have a particularly high amount of stored sun energy that is transferred to us when we eat them. The more light a food can store, the healthier it is. According to Dr. Gabriel Cousens, many diseases that perplex doctors, due to lab tests showing no disease, are a result of a drop in the electrical potential at the cellular level. He states that raw foods restore the electrical potential of the cells by rejuvenating the life force and health of the organism. Raw, living foods affect every cell in our bodies by restoring their microelectrical potential and their overall ability to function optimally. Cousens also states that biophotons seem to be an important part of regulating every metabolic process in the body. He says that the more biophoton rich food we ingest, the better the intra- and extracellular communication will be and therefore the better our health will be. It makes sense then that the lack of biophotons in processed and cooked foods is one more reason that they have such a negative impact on our overall wellbeing. It also makes sense that people look so much more alive and vibrant after ten days on the Challenge. I had one Challenger tell me that she visited her doctor after taking the Challenge and he said, "I don't know what you are doing but you look healthier and younger and you should keep doing whatever you are doing!"

Since writing the first edition of this book, I have become aware that pure therapeutic grade essential oils have the highest energy potential of anything we can put into our bodies. I now add essential oils (only **Young Living brand** as not all are safe for internal consumption) to my smoothies for even more life giving and disease fighting potential. Young Living essential oils have been shown to raise the energy potential even with

---

[18] Mercola, Dr. Joseph. How Drinking More Spring or Filtered Water Can Improve Every Facet of Your Health. Retrieved from http://www.mercola.com/article/water.htm

[19] Mercola, Dr. Joseph (2002, August 21). McDonald's and Biophoton Deficiency. Retrieved from http://articles.mercola.com/sites/articles/archive/2002/08/21/biophoton.aspx

[20] Cousens, Dr. Gabriel, MD. *Conscious Eating*, North Atlantic Books, Berkeley, CA 2000. 571-572

[21] Cousens, Dr. Gabriel, MD. *Conscious Eating*, North Atlantic Books, Berkeley, CA 2000. 577-578

inhalation affecting the emotions on a positive level as well.

Polyphenols. As for the fruit portion of the smoothie, berries are important ingredients. Strawberries, blackberries, blueberries and cranberries contain ellagic acid and a large amount of polyphenols. Polyphenols are a more recently discovered group of phytochemicals that act as antioxidants. They are immune boosting and cancer fighting. These powerful compounds are also found in red wine, green tea, and chocolate.

As you can see, green smoothies contribute to our overall health and well being. "Unfortunately many of our health-care problems are self-inflicted; two-thirds of Americans are now overweight and one-third are obese. Most of the diseases that kill us and account for about 70% of all health-care spending—heart disease, cancer, stroke, diabetes and obesity—are mostly preventable through proper diet, exercise, not smoking, minimal alcohol consumption and other healthy lifestyle choices.

"Recent scientific and medical evidence shows that a diet consisting of foods that are plant-based, nutrient dense, and low-fat will help prevent and often reverse most degenerative diseases that kill us and are expensive to treat. We should be able to live largely disease-free lives until we are well into our 90s and even past 100 years of age."

Although I firmly believe that eating a certain amount of high quality animal fat and protein is necessary for vibrant health, for a time while cleansing, it is beneficial to take a break from eating animal-based foods. I also believe that low fat does not mean eating low-fat foods, but rather finding the right amount of healthy fat for your particular metabolic type and not over-doing it OR being afraid to eat it. Not only are green smoothies plant-based, nutrient dense and low fat, they are alkalizing. What does this mean for you? Much scientific evidence points to the fact that disease cannot thrive in an alkaline environment. Most foods eaten in the Standard American Diet (SAD) are acid forming. When we eat acid forming food, the environment inside our bodies becomes acidic, creating a perfect environment for bacteria, viruses, fungus, cancer, etc. to thrive. An acid condition in the body has also been shown to cause the body to retain water in order to dilute the acids. This causes weight gain and fat retention. Often when people begin The Green Smoothie Challenge, the first thing they notice is that they urinate a LOT. I believe this is due in part to the fact that your body is releasing the retained water as you ingest the nutrient dense, alkaline forming green smoothies. It is also a good sign that detoxification is occurring. Another possibility is that one may be eating foods they are allergic to and retaining water. When those foods are eliminated, it is possible to

---

[22] Murray, Michael, ND, The Encyclopedia of Healing Foods, Atria Books, New York, 2005.

[23] Mackey, John, co-founder and CEO of Whole Foods Market, Inc., 'The Whole Foods Alternative to Obama Care,' The Wall Street Journal online, August 11, 2009, http://online.wsj.com/articles/SB10001424052970204251404574342170072865070

release a lot of weight very quickly due to the excess water being released.

What Can a Green Smoothie Include?

The only contents of a green smoothie should be fruit, vegetable fruits, green, leafy and non-starchy vegetables, herbs, and water. Green leafy vegetables are the dark green ones. They include things like collard greens, kale, dandelion greens, spinach, romaine lettuce, baby spring greens, arugula, radicchio, beet greens, carrot tops, bok choy, wheat grass, mustard greens and radish tops. Try using any of the red, green or purple lettuce leaves too. You may use vegetable fruits such as cucumbers, bell peppers, avocados, tomatoes, zucchini and the like. Add herbs such as celery, fennel, ginger, parsley or cilantro. Lemon and lime give a nutritional punch and add a refreshing flavor. These are both cleansing fruits that will add to your weight releasing success. I like to use half of a lemon or lime, with some or all of the peel. The white flesh of these citrusy gems and the peel are full of key nutrients.

Do not use starchy vegetables such as carrots, beets, corn, potatoes, peas or any other vegetables that are considered starchy. I also like to add broccoli stems (skin trimmed off), but not the florets as they can cause abdominal discomfort or bloating in many people. Feel free to use lightly steamed broccoli if that appeals to you. You may also add onion, garlic, radishes, lemon and lime or even coconut.

I enjoy the young Thai coconuts, which have a white outer husk and are commonly found in Asian markets. You can use coconut water in place of plain water in your smoothie. The water inside this tropical nut very closely resembles human blood plasma having the highest content of electrolytes of any food found in nature. It is the perfect sports drink. In fact, according to the American Journal of Emergency Medicine, coconut water has been used successfully as a "short term intravenous hydration fluid." Proper hydration is energizing making this natural beverage a perfect way to start your day. Use organic young Thai coconuts when possible. You can also find organic versions of coconut water or coconut juice in your health food store. To super-charge your coconut water, you can ferment it. **Learn how at www.youtube.com**.

My favorite herbs to add are aloe, parsley, fennel and cilantro. I also prefer ginger in my smoothies. Go tour the produce aisle in your local natural grocery store and see what you can find. There are so many options and combinations. Of course, you are also free to simply follow my recipes if you are not comfortable experimenting.

For the more adventurous green smoothie fan, another interesting addition is wild

---

[24] The Intravenous Use of Coconut Water. The American Journal of Emergency Medicine, Volume 18, Issue 1, Pages 108-111. D.Campbell-Falck, T.Thomas, T.Falck, N.Tutuo, K.Clem

edible leaves if you know which ones are safe to eat. Consider taking a wild edibles class from a local teacher to learn about the free wild herbs and greens you can add to your smoothies. Just be careful to add these slowly and sparingly, as they are highly nutritious and have potent medicinal properties.

Fruit digests very quickly. When mixed with foods other than green, leafy vegetables, vegetable fruits or non-starchy vegetables, your stomach will let the fruit sit while it digests the other foods it finds there. This will cause the fruit to begin to ferment, which creates gas. You may use any fruits you like, but stay away from starchy veggies. This will enable the greens and fruit to be digested fully and efficiently, allowing your body to absorb their full nutritional benefits.

I do not recommend using certain cruciferous vegetables such as broccoli, cauliflower or cabbage in the smoothies. In their raw, unfermented state, these veggies can cause abdominal discomfort, to put it nicely. Feel free to use them steamed, if you choose to add them to your smoothies.

It is important to only use *dark* green leafy vegetables. Iceberg lettuce, though possibly tempting to use, should not be included in your smoothie because it lacks the chlorophyll and other important nutrients only found in dark varieties of leafy greens. Experiment with bok choy, spinach, baby greens, wheat grass, carrot tops, radish tops, arugula, radicchio, kale, collards, chard, dandelion greens, sprouts—used sparingly, endive, escarole, beet greens, romaine lettuce, lamb's quarters, leeks, mustard greens and any other interesting greens you can find including all dark green or purple lettuces.

Organic produce is superior and important to use during The Challenge. I will go into more detail about this a little later.

Using low-glycemic fruits will increase your healing speed as well as your weight-loss. Low glycemic means low sugar, so the less sugar the fruit has, the more weight you will release. Low-glycemic fruits include grapefruit, lemon, lime, cherries, strawberries, cranberries, raspberries, goji berries and blueberries. Moderate glycemic fruits include peaches, oranges, pears, apples, pomegranate and plums. The high-sugar content fruits are apricots, melons, kiwi, mango, papaya, pineapple, banana, date, fig, raisins and grapes.

Tap water is not recommended for use. Use purified water or spring water.

---

[25] Cousens, Gabriel, MD, Rainbow Green Live-Food Cuisine, North Atlantic Books, Berkeley, CA, 2003.

How Long Will My Smoothie Keep?

It is always optimal to drink your smoothie the same day you mix it. However, if you have some left over and wish to consume it the following day, that if just fine. When you break down the fibers of the fruits and vegetables and expose them to air, they do begin to oxidize and quickly lose enzymes and nutrition. Ingesting them sooner is best although they will last up to three days. For storage purposes, simply add the leftover portion to a glass jar immediately after blending and fill the jar to the top with your smoothie, cap it with a lid and place it directly in the refrigerator. This will help to prevent oxidation, as air won't be able to get to it if it is filled to the rim.

---

[26] Boutenko, Victoria, Green Smoothie Revolution, North Atlantic Books, Berkeley, CA 2009

CHAPTER 2
Frequently Asked Questions

It is unlikely that any damage will be caused by consuming only fruits and vegetables for a period of two weeks or less. Not only is it safe to eat a large amount of plant foods, it may well add years to your life. Blended fruits and vegetables are cleansing, so there is a possibility that you may experience a detoxification reaction as your body cleanses. With the more toxic buildup that exists in your system, the more chance you have of this reaction occurring. It is essentially a withdrawal symptom.

How does toxic buildup occur? When the body's process of cell regeneration and rebuilding begins to slow down, we age. "This slowdown is caused by the accumulation of waste products in the tissues which interferes with the nourishment of the cells." A sluggish metabolism due to poor eating habits and lack of exercise, along with constipation, causes the body to retain toxic waste that accumulates in our tissues. When this occurs, it interferes with the proper nourishment of our cells, and they begin to deteriorate. Our cells are in a constant cycle of growth and development followed by dying off and being replaced. It is when more cells are dying off than are growing or our new cells are being created with less-than-optimal nutrition, that we begin to age which is basically our body moving towards death, breaking down. We have some control over this process in regards to our lifestyle. We can assist in the process of growing healthy, nourished cells or we can contribute to the deterioration of the cells through behaviors that promote their break down.

If we have mostly chosen a lifestyle that promotes toxic buildup such as eating many processed and overly cooked foods, over-consumption of alcohol, lack of exercise, high stress levels, etc., then we may experience a cleansing reaction as the toxins begin to exit the system. This would possibly involve getting a headache, body aches, a cold or the flu, being extra tired, breaking out in a rash, a cold or something similar. The best

---

[27] Airola, Dr. Paavo, PhD, How to Keep Slim, Healthy and Young with Juice Fasting, Health Plus Publishers, Sherwood, OR, 1971.

[28] Airola, Paavo, How to Keep Slim, Healthy and Young with Juice Fasting, Health Plus Publishers, Sherwood, OR, 1971

thing to do in this circumstance is to let it work itself out. There is no reason to panic or stop The Challenge. If you are able, avoid taking medication to stop these symptoms. Once this stage passes, you will feel amazing. Listen to your body. If you have concerns, see a qualified health professional who is accustomed to guiding people through a body cleanse such as this. It is important to check with your physician or natural health care provider before beginning The Challenge to make sure this is safe for you. If you are currently taking medications, it is of utmost importance to get cleared by your doctor before taking on The Green Smoothie Challenge.

A note from Dr. Donato: "If the person following the diet is a female, over 40, and has had children, and has lost a lot of weight in a short time, this is risk for gall stone problems. I have had probably five cases. Three had to have their gall bladders taken out, and one ended up in ICU."

"Those students who had gall stone attacks experienced it within ten weeks. One person experienced it approximately nine months into an all-raw, no animal products, vegan lifestyle. It can also definitely happen to men, and it does not have to fit in those parameters I mentioned earlier. In the raw-food, vegan lifestyle, weight-loss and health improvement are usually predictable. But when it comes to massive detox symptoms (e.g. gall stone attack), they are unpredictable. Most people will do fine. The ones who are more at risk are the ones who have pre-existing health conditions like diabetes, heart disease, fibromyalgia, cancer, etc. Also at risk are those who are taking several prescription medications. People who are on Coumadin will have to first talk to their doctor about going "green" before starting. When the body becomes healthy, the drugs can do damage. That's why these people need to be monitored by health professionals. The average "healthy" middle-aged person will likely do well. I'm talking about a high raw vegan diet that is greater than 85% raw over an extended period of time."

"A 10-day green smoothie challenge is probably too short to induce massive detox. Most likely, it won't happen (has not happened to my students), but it's not impossible. I know I am not being exact. It is not a science! And yes it is fairly safe for most people."

Who Should Take The Challenge?

It is a commonly accepted opinion that it is safe for a person to take on a juice fast for ten to fourteen days at home. Of course, if there are health concerns involved, a doctor's recommendation must be obtained, and it is always a good idea to have a physical

---

[29] Airola, Dr. Paavo O, How to Keep Slim, Healthy and Young with Juice Fasting, Health Plus Publishers, Sherwood, Oregon, 1971

examination before taking on such an endeavor. For the general population, the 10-day Challenge is a safe and effective way to eliminate damaging and addicting foods from the diet in order to gain energy and vitality, as well as release weight. Remember it is always in your best interest to seek the advice of your doctor before ever making drastic changes to your diet.

If you are taking pharmaceutical drugs, it is prudent to consult your physician before embarking on the Challenge as high levels of brassica vegetables may possibly have certain drug interactions. Instead, make vegetable soups or use my 'Daily Sunshine Smoothie' recipe or my 'Thyroid Safe' smoothie recipe; neither use dark leafy greens. As a general rule, you can replace dark, leafy greens in any recipe with celery, cucumber, zucchini or any other vegetable fruits. Just stay clear of the starchy vegetables.

Dark, leafy green vegetables are high in vitamin K, which is known to be a natural blood thinner. Those taking blood-thinning medication should refrain from drinking green smoothies that include dark, leafy green vegetables unless they have specific permission from their physician. You can use cucumbers, celery and zucchini instead of dark leafy greens as your vegetable base.

People who are more than 10% below their suggested weight should not take The Challenge. Those who have an eating disorder must consult with their physician before taking on The Challenge, as it is never good for your health to binge and purge.

People whose thyroid function is low or are on thyroid medication may want to customize their Challenge to avoid eating raw, cruciferous vegetables. Members of the Brassica family have the potential to block the formation of thyroid hormone and should be avoided by people with low thyroid function or low iodine. This is due to the goitrogenic (anti-thyroid) effect of these vegetables in their raw form. If you have thyroid concerns, eating fermented cruciferous vegetables may be the preferred choice, as they are not known to impact the thyroid. Feel free to make brassica-free smoothies or simply avoid the cruciferous vegetables, which are kale, collard greens, broccoli, cabbage, brussel sprouts, kohlrabi, cauliflower, mustard greens, bok choy, arugula, radishes, rutabaga, turnips and daikon. You will find my thyroid safe smoothie as well as my 'Daily Sunshine' smoothie recipe in Chapter 6. I've found it is best for you to use cucumbers, zucchini and celery as your vegetable base while adding in ½ an avocado for the fat which will support your thyroid.

There is also the possibility that certain other fruits and vegetables can have the same affect. These include carrots, peaches, strawberries and spinach. There is less risk of this occurring if one's diet is high in iodine rich foods such as Dulse or kelp. It is important to note that when fermented, cruciferous vegetables do not have the goitrogenic effect. I always add sea vegetables to my fermented vegetables, which adds even more protection. If you begin to feel very cold and tired or your skin is extremely dry, you may be experiencing the effect of eating too many raw cruciferous vegetables. Try going off of them for a time while adding iodine-rich foods to your diet and see if the symptoms improve.

Many people are not properly diagnosed for low thyroid function. The symptoms for low thyroid are many and include, brittle nails, cold hands and feet, cold intolerance, depression, difficulty swallowing, dry skin, elevated cholesterol, essential hypertension, eyelid swelling, fatigue, hair loss, hoarseness, inability to concentrate, infertility, irritability, menstrual irregularities, muscles cramps, muscle weakness, nervousness, poor memory, puffy eyes, slower heartbeat, throat pain, weight gain. If you are experiencing many of these symptoms, chances are that you have low thyroid. In order to be certain, you can purchase a basal temperature thermometer. Check your temperature beginning on the second day of menstruation (for women). Place the thermometer next to your bed at night, and in the morning before getting out of bed take your temperature under the arm pit for ten minutes. If the average temperature for three days in a row is under 97.8, low thyroid is a good possibility. If you suspect low thyroid even though your thyroid tests appear normal, you can find treatment information in the following excellent books: *Hypothyroidism: the Unsuspected Illness*, by Broda O. Barnes, MD and Overcoming Thyroid Disorders, by David Brownstein, MD. You can find my thyroid friendly smoothie recipe in Chapter 7. I recommend that every reader educate themselves about taking iodine. Please read *Iodine: Why You Need it, Why You Can't Live Without It*.

Please listen to your body and do not try to out-do your friends. Competition in this way does not have a health enhancing effect on the body and is not a proper motivation for cleansing.

It may be best for you to only try this for one day. You can then begin to change your diet gradually and then do The Challenge for more days as you increase your level of health slowly. The key is finding what works best for you personally. This is certainly not a perfection test and what works for one person does not necessarily work for another. We are looking for lifestyle improvement, so I invite you to focus on being thrilled with every improvement instead of being upset about areas you have not yet improved! Consider adding more healthy foods to your current diet instead of taking away unhealthy foods.

If your motivation for taking The Challenge is to enhance your health, get your energy back and keep a slim physique while living a healthy lifestyle in general, then by all means, you are the right person to take on this experience.

---

[30] Brownstein, David, M.D., Iodine, Why You Need it, Why You Can't Live Without it, 4th Edition, Medical Alternatives Press, West Bloomfield, MI, 2009.

> **Caution:** If you find yourself continually wanting to cleanse and then eating a diet full of processed or less than optimal foods or even just over-eating in between cleanses, it may be a good time to take a look at this pattern in a very non-judgmental, self-compassionate way. Our tendency, mine anyway, can be to stop and take a look at a pattern we have, and think it is wrong and we are bad. Instead, simply ask yourself if you need to find more balance in your relationship to food. If the answer is yes, seek out ways to do this successfully. I offer coaching to help people find this balance. It is so normal to get off track in this area and getting back on track is very attainable. If you feel extra support would be helpful, feel free to **book a complimentary appointment with me, at www.mariarippo.com**.

Are you cleansing to be kind to your body or are you doing it often and to release the weight you gain when not taking the Challenge? I recommend only taking the Challenge twice a year. More often than this would signal to me that there may be underlying issues that need some love and attention. I know I was cleansing far too often for a time. What I learned to do was to realize that this pattern held an important message for me. You see, in the past, I would be very hard on myself when I realized areas that needed attention. It was freeing for me to realize that when I was acting in a way that I wanted to see change, I only needed to look for the message in it, find how part of me was benefitting from the behavior and be OK realizing that it is normal that we act out less-than-optimal behaviors at times in order to meet underlying needs we have that we are typically unaware of. It took me a long while to be accepting of this in myself. Once I became aware of how part of me was benefitting from the negative behavior, I was able to make new choices for my life.

You will need a good dose of perseverance to complete The Challenge. According to the Character Counts program, **perseverance** is sticking to a task even when it's difficult. It's striving and pushing yourself, sometimes beyond the limits you thought you had (when giving up would seem an easier option) in order to push for the finish line.

The American Heritage Dictionary defines perseverance as "adherence to a course of action, belief or purpose without giving way; steadfastness." When we persevere, when we stick to our commitments, miracles happen, we are transformed and strengthened in

---

[31] Character Counts Web site http://charactercounts.org/lesson-plans/character-education-lesson.php?id=11

[32] The American Heritage Dictionary, Second College Edition, Houghton Mifflin Company, Boston, MA, 1985.

a way that gives us a totally new resolve, a new lease on life. You owe it to yourself to stick to this. You can do it and you will be amazed at the results when you do. When you work beyond your resistance and cravings, miracles begin to happen.

Why Do a Cleanse?

In order for the body to be able to cleanse, we must stop adding junk to our system. Junk includes any food that does not *add* health to your body. For example, white flour acts like glue in the colon, clogging it up and causing waste to build up. It, along with refined sugar, increases insulin levels causing the body to store fat. The combination of sugar, fat and salt can have an addictive effect on many people, causing them to want more and more and to never feel satisfied by it. Processed food producers know this all too well and actually formulate their foods scientifically to have this addictive effect on you. "The neurons in the brain that are stimulated by taste and other properties of highly palatable food are part of the opioid circuitry, which is the body's primary pleasure system. The 'opioids,' also known as endorphins, are chemicals produced in the brain that have rewarding effects similar to drugs such as morphine and heroin. It has also been found that "the opioids produced by eating high-fat, high-sugar foods can relieve pain or stress and calm us down. At least in the short run they make us feel better. It's no wonder that we eat foods that are less-than-optimal for our health. With the amount of stress people are living with (at least 25% more anxiety than in past generations), food is an easy way to get fast relief. The problem shows up after the fact, but often we don't associate our ill-health with the food choices we make.

Gluten is another important food to eliminate from the diet as it can cause damage and inflammation to the intestinal tract as well as weight gain in many people.

A detoxifying cleanse enables the colon to excrete waste and bacterial or parasitic build-up. It is common to have an overgrowth of yeast in the colon (Candida Albicans), as well. All of these factors can wreak havoc on your state of health. Taking enzymes, probiotics and cleaning out the colon through a diet of green smoothies will give your colon the extra boost it needs to become healthy. Cleaning out the colon can have a tremendous healing impact on the body. You are also giving your digestive system a break, which enables your body to focus its energy on rebuilding and purifying itself. In order for our bodies to function optimally, our blood and organs must be clean. If your colon is congested, your body will not get as much benefit from the smoothies. You absorb hundreds of times more nutrients when your colon is clear. Taking The Challenge helps to clear the colon, enabling the body to absorb more nutrition.

---

[33] Kessler, David A. The End of Overeating. Taking Control of the Insatiable American Appetite. New York: Rodale Books, 2009. Print.

[34] Ibid

34

If you have difficulty releasing weight, toxic buildup may be the culprit. Nutritionist Natalia Rose, in her book, **The Raw Food Detox Diet**, uses a simple equation to illustrate the importance of detoxification for weight loss:

Waste = Weight

She explains that waste matter in the body is the fundamental source of the excess weight in your body. Enzymes and proper hydration are the mechanisms that your body uses to renew your cells. Besides doing a juice fast or blended food cleanse, Rose also recommends colon hydrotherapy (colonics), rebounding (light bouncing on a small trampoline), dry brush massage, deep breathing, breaking a sweat and getting plenty of sunshine, along with eating a cleansing diet.

Ann Louise Gittleman, PhD, CNS, explains that "if you have trouble losing weight or maintaining your ideal weight, even if you regulate eating and exercise regularly, you should definitely consider whether a toxic colon or liver are your problem."

Colon hydrotherapy (colonic) is one of the most effective ways to thoroughly cleanse the colon. Once you have begun a cleansing diet, if you are not evacuating at least twelve inches of fecal matter per day, you most likely have buildup that is preventing proper elimination. Rose suggests that another way to tell if you have buildup is to look at your abdomen after urinating first thing in the morning. If you can pull your belly button in close to your spine then you may not have a lot of buildup. On the other hand, if you can't, you do have buildup. During a colonic, water will flow gently in and out of your colon through a tube as your therapist massages it to help release built-up matter. An experienced colon hydrotherapist will allow for a pleasant experience that is gentle, comfortable and modest.

Natural health pioneer and author of **Tissue Cleansing Through Bowel Management**, Nutritionist, Bernard Jensen, DC, explains that toxic material decaying away in the sigmoid colon is a good place for degenerative diseases to get started. If you eat three meals a day and only eliminate once in five days, imagine how much waste is left behind! Jensen states that the primary causes of constipation are lack of proper nutrition, ignoring the need to eliminate, lack of exercise which tones the colon, emotional and mental distress, extrinsic poisons, medications, and lack of adequate hydration.

Jensen also discusses Henrig's law of cure, which states that "diseases are cured from

---

[35] Rose, Natalia, *The Raw Food Detox Diet*, Harper Collins Publishers, Inc. New York, NY, 2006.

[36] Gittleman, Ann Louise,PhD, CNS, *The Fast Track Detox Diet*, Broadway Books, NY, 2005 and *The Living Beauty Detox Program*, Harper Collins, San Fransisco, 2000.

within out, from the head down, and in reverse order as their symptoms first appeared in the body. No disease can exist without toxic material in the body, so the first step toward remission is detoxification."

Using a reputable colon hydrotherapist is of utmost importance if you choose to do colon hydrotherapy. I have linked to a list of reputable clinics below. You will want to speak to the therapist before your first appointment so you know what to expect. Check out Natalia Rose's Colon Therapy Directory at **http://www.detoxtheworld.com**.

What Do I Need to Get Started?

In order to get started, you will need a good dose of perseverance, the shopping list included in this book, a blender, containers or glass jars to hold your smoothies, various herbal teas and the optional extra supplements I will discuss.

A high-speed blender is the preferred option. I prefer the **Blendtec™ 3 horsepower blender**. You could use a regular blender, but you may end up with a chunky consistency requiring that you chew the smoothie before swallowing. If necessary, start with the blender you already have and then decide if you need a more powerful one after you have made the commitment to drink green smoothies on a daily basis. Read through this entire guide before you begin. It is very important that you know what to expect, especially from both the emotional as well as the physical standpoint.

Consider taking a "before" picture. Take one full body, and one close-up of your face. This will enable you to see the physical changes that take place. Many times, you will see a big difference in the way your eyes appear. We tend to hold toxins in the eye area.

Write out your plan for this Challenge and the 'Why' statement you will develop in Chapter 3. Place a 10-day calendar on your bathroom mirror and cross off each day as it passes. You'll find this calendar, along with other resources for your Challenge at **www.mariarippo.com/your-green-smoothie-challenge-tool-kit.html**.

Consider using a special glass for drinking your smoothie. I prefer a martini glass because of its celebratory feel. This is a celebration of life, of vitality, of success. Make a toast to your efforts every time you drink!

You'll use the shopping list I have included in Chapter 6 for the entire 10-day experience for your trip to the produce aisle. It is broken into the first five days and the second five days. Only shop for five days at a time, as this will ensure your produce is fresh! The list

---

[37] Jensen, Bernard, DC, Nutritionist, *Tissue Cleansing Through Bowel Management*, Escondido, CA Bernard Jensen Publishing, 1981.

corresponds to the first ten green smoothie recipes you will find in Chapter 7.

How Important Are Supplements?

Whether or not you continue to take your current supplements during The Challenge is up to you. I prefer not take vitamin supplements when I cleanse. In this section, I discuss some supplements that will enhance the cleansing process and are a helpful addition to The Challenge. If you are taking medications, make sure to check with your physician about doing a cleanse while on medications.

What About Green Superfoods?

Spirulina, chlorella and **Klammath Lake blue-green algae** are green superfoods. If you are feeling the urge to gag at the thought of tasting something like this, rest assured, these products are available in a convenient capsule form to swallow without ever tasting them. It is an amazing pick-me-up between smoothies. An optimum choice is **E3Live™**. I use a green powder every morning called **Vitality Super Green from bodyecology.com**. It is gut healing, mineralizing and alkalizing. I add the juice from ½ a lemon to the powder and drink it with water.

Green superfoods are excellent sources of chlorophyll. Spirulina is a rich source of iron, beta carotene, calcium, protein, phytonutrients, enzymes and antioxidants. It is close to 70% protein. No other food contains such a high amount of this all-important nutrient. Because of its superior amounts of chlorophyll, spirulina is a strong blood purifier and builder. If you are an athlete or exercise regularly, this is an ideal supplement to give you extra protein, without adding calories.

You may want to take up to three tablespoons of spirulina per day. Start slowly and observe how it makes you feel. Increase the amount gradually, finding the appropriate dosage for your body.

Klammath Lake blue-green algae is known as a super brain food. It has anti-inflamatory properties, the ability to strengthen the immune system and contains potent anti-viral qualities. It is a rich source of chlorophyll, which cleanses the blood. It is high in beta carotene, B-complex vitamins, fatty acids, enzymes, essential amino acids and nucleic acids, which are essential for growth and repair. The essential amino acid make-up of blue-green algae is almost identical to that of human blood.

Chlorella, according to nutritionist and superfood expert David Wolfe, supports the function of the brain and liver, improves digestion and elimination, helps regenerate the body, detoxifies the blood, protects against radiation, relieves inflammation, supports healthy weight loss, enhances immune function and accelerates the healing process. Chlorella is also commonly used to remove toxic heavy metals from the tissues. If that is not enough to convince you to use this superfood, you might consider taking it to improve your decision-making abilities!

These three superfoods would be an excellent addition to any diet. It is especially important to start small and work up with these. Power Organics™, the maker of Klammath Power 3, recommends taking one capsule per day and working up to two to ten per day.

Probiotics

Within the human body there is an ecosystem made up of bacteria. The colon (mostly the large intestine) is the place where the bacterial ecosystem must be balanced in order to experience true health. There happen to be over seven hundred types of harmful bacteria and only twenty types that are beneficial. The ironic fact is that 85% of the bacteria in our colon must be the beneficial type in order to have a healthy balance. It is very easy for this essential balance to get off track, and when it does, serious health problems can arise. A few factors that contribute to the imbalance are:

- using antibiotics
- consuming refined sugars
- consuming processed carbohydrates
- drinking tap water treated with chlorine and laden with residues of antibiotics
- regularly consuming alcohol.

An imbalance in good-to-bad bacteria results in toxemia, which is toxic blood. A good and reputable source of probiotics can help to implant millions of good bacteria inside the colon and bring the proper balance back to the intestines. There are a few ways to accomplish this. One is by taking a potent probiotic supplement. Creating a proper colon ecology is the number one way to improve your health. Most people have 85% bad bacteria and yeast in their colon and 15% good bacteria. This ratio needs to be turned around in order to experience optimum health. By creating an environment of 85% good bacteria, you will notice improved digestion and absorption of vitamins and minerals leading to increased energy, enhanced immune function and improved overall wellbeing. According to Chinese Medicine, 80% of our immune system is in our digestive tract. Current scientific research also confirms this fact. In addition, "A healthy and happy digestive system may help you keep your waistline slim and trim. And recent

---

[38] Wolfe, David, Superfoods, North Atlantic Books, Berkeley, CA 2009.

scientific studies also show that supplementing with probiotics may help reduce fat. By taking a probiotic supplement you will increase nutrient absorption, improve the ability to eliminate, and strengthen the immune system. The best way I have found to recolonize the intestinal tract with beneficial bacteria is the Rejuviflora System by Interplexus. This is a five-month recolonization program and the investment is only $122. I can't think of a better way to spend this money that in giving your body the gift of balancing the flora. For a special discount on this product, **email me for more information: maria@mariarippo.com**.

Digestive Enzymes

Imagine journeying to the fountain of youth. Just take a dip, and *poof*! You are young and healthy again. What if I told you that you could begin the process of becoming more youthful and healthy today? You can. Would you like to know how? Read on.

In addition to balancing the flora in your intestines, eating food that is full of **enzymes** will do just that. It will make you look and feel younger and healthier and help to prevent and fight cancer and other sicknesses. Enzymes are vital for life. They are involved in every process of the body that is necessary to sustain life. Without enzymes, there is no life. As I mentioned previously, they are the construction crew of the body. (Remember, proteins are the building blocks.)

In order to supercharge your Challenge and avoid experiencing the feelings of ill due to detox, you can add more enzymes to your system through supplementation. This will speed up your cleansing process, as well as help you to feel great and look younger faster than if you did not choose to take them. Taking an enzyme supplement will help you absorb more nutrients and receive the maximum benefits of your Challenge.

Can I Exercise While Taking The Challenge?

Exercising while on The Challenge is very important. The best types of exercises are brisk walking, yoga (not power or hot yoga) and rebounding, which is bouncing on a mini-trampoline. According to nutritionist Natalia Rose, author of *The Raw Food Detox Diet*, rebounding "is possibly the single best exercise on the planet. Rebounding literally squeezes the waste matter from our cells as we bounce effortlessly for just a short time. It is ideal for circulation and great for toning the whole body." Rebounding is the only

---

[39] *European Journal of Clinical Nutrition*, June 2010, Volume 64, Number 6, Pages 636-643 "Regulation of abdominal adiposity by probiotics (Lactobacillus gasseri SBT2055) in adults with obese tendencies in a randomized controlled trial." Authors: Y. Kadooka, M. Sato, K. Imaizumi, A. Ogawa, K. Ikuyama, Y. Akai, M. Okano, M. Kagoshima, T. Tsuchida

[40] Rose, Natalia, *The Raw Food Detox Diet*, Harper Collins Publishers, Inc. New York, NY, 2006.

way I know of to cleanse the lymphatic system. A sluggish lymphatic system is often a leading cause of cellulite on the thigh and buttocks area. If you do not currently exercise regularly, start small. Take a fifteen-minute walk today and gradually increase your time over the next ten days. It is always best not to just dive right in and make yourself take an hour walk when you are not accustomed to exercising. This is a recipe for possible burnout or injury.

One thing that I like to remember when I begin something is to look at the improvement I've made. Look at how I have upgraded my eating or my exercising by one step. I used to tend to be upset that I was not at my goal until I realized that attaining a goal is a matter of taking many small, consistent steps to get there. The Chinese philosopher, Lau-tzu said, "A journey of a thousand miles begins with a single step." So, if your baby steps are bringing you closer to your goal, then you are doing great. Before you know it, you will have attained the prize! Focus on what you are now doing that is better than before, rather than on what you are not doing yet.

If you are an athlete and choose to continue exercising heavily during The Challenge, here is what Dr. Donato has to say:

> "In the beginning, just losing weight can make a person feel great and energetic but over time if the caloric intake remains low in someone who is expending tremendous energy by means of exercise, the end result will be low energy storage, and ultimately catabolic process (your body consuming its own tissue). The person will feel tired and less motivated and could eventually run the risk of contracting a disease of deficiency. But for short-term, continuing heavier exercise while taking The Challenge is probably acceptable for athletes."

It is important as an athlete to support your body through caloric intake. Listen to your body and eat extra soaked nuts or avocados and take extra spirulina, chlorella and blue-green algae, if necessary. Many people have had to stop taking The Challenge because they are simply exercising too heavily while not eating enough calories, especially fat and protein. I tend to take a break from heavy exercise when I cleanse. Exercise is stressful to the body and stress is acid forming. Part of the purpose of eating so many greens is to bring your body into a less acidic state. Disease thrives in an acidic environment. Taking a small break from intense exercise will give your body a rest and actually make you stronger in the end. I do not recommend heavy weight lifting while on The Challenge. Consider giving the gift of a change of pace and a rest to your body. Get outside, take a brisk walk and do some deep stretching instead. Yoga and rebounding are the perfect exercise while cleansing. Stay away from power yoga or

---

[41] Gittleman, Ann Louise, *The Fat Flush Plan,* McGraw Hill, 2002)

[42] Donato, Miven, e-mail correspondence, December 1 and 2, 2009.

intense hot yoga for now because that will take so much out of you it may cause more harm than good if all you are consuming is smoothies.

If you do choose to continue exercising heavily while taking The Challenge, you can read about The Challenge option called the *Performance Enhancer* in Chapter 4.

What Else Can I Do to Help My Body Cleanse Even More?

Hydrotherapy in the shower! Simply take a hot shower and at the end, turn the water from hot to cold, to hot and back to cold. This is a simple and free way to stimulate the metabolism and the immune system. It also increases blood flow, which stimulates the circulatory system and brings extra oxygen and nutrients to your cells and tissues. Also, consider installing a **water purifier** in your shower.

Dry Brush Massage. The skin is our largest organ and is a major eliminatory organ. A simple way to increase toxic elimination through the skin as well as rejuvenating the skin itself is by using a dry brush to massage the skin of the entire body before bathing. A dry brush for this purpose is available in almost any pharmacy or health food store. Make sure the brush is made of natural bristles and has a long handle. Start with your feet and legs, then hands and arms, abdomen and back, chest and neck. Use a circular motion. Do not use a nylon or **synthetic bristle brush** as this may damage your skin.

Water with Apple Cider Vinegar and Good Salt.

Simply add one tablespoon **raw apple cider vinegar** plus ⅛ teaspoon **Celtic Sea** or **Himalayan** salt to one of your water bottles each day. This is cleansing, hydrating and immune enhancing.

Troubleshooting: What if I Just Have to Eat?

If you come to a point where you feel you would like to stop The Challenge, there are a few things to try. First, know this feeling is normal and that it *will* pass. Try making yourself an extra yummy smoothie or have a fresh green juice. Have a few celery sticks, carrots or an apple. Make a batch of my strawberry ice cream in Chapter 6. Whip up a "Heavenly Chocolate Shake" also in Chapter 6. Have a handful of raw nuts or seeds. Drink a refreshing cup of tea. Make some of my guacamole and use carrots, celery, cucumbers, bell peppers or jicama for the chips. For the first few days, this will really help to curb your hunger. Look forward to days five and following as your amazing weight loss results and feelings of high energy will begin to outweigh the longing to eat those less-than-optimal, but tempting foods you are accustomed to consuming

---

[43] Airola, Paavo O., *How to Keep Slim, Healthy and Young with Juice Fasting*, Health Plus Publishers, Sherwood, OR 1971.

41

regularly. The most helpful tool I have found in times of intense temptation is focus on the choices I can make in the moment that will help me attain my goals instead of focusing on the choices that will keep me from my goals and tempt me to feel I have failed.

The other helpful tool is to stop, get in a comfortable position, take some deep breaths and imagine the new you walking along a sunny beach, full of energy and vitality, skipping, swimming, anything that you would love to be doing. *See* yourself how want to be. As Earl Nightengale so famously said, "the strangest secret in the world is that we become what we think about."

One common tendency that we have when we struggle is to try *not to struggle*. We may begin to obsess over the foods we have temporarily chosen to avoid. If you try to ignore the fact you are struggling, the feeling may persist. Instead, try saying to yourself:

"Self, this really is a tough Challenge. Even though I really want to eat some foods that are not part of The Challenge right now, I fully and completely love and accept myself anyway. And even though I want to throw in the towel and pig out, I completely love and accept myself. Even though I feel like cheating and eating whatever I want, I still deeply love and accept myself. I am very hungry and not feeling comfortable. I have such strong cravings and I'd really like to eat some food that is not part of this Challenge. I know it would taste so good and the texture would melt in my mouth. It would give me so much satisfaction. It would feel so good. It would really make me happy. But I have made a positive choice for myself. I am giving my body the gift of a cleanse. My energy level is going to soar. My cravings will become less. I will feel so light, and will feel so strong and empowered when I have stuck to my commitment. I choose to stick to my commitment, because it's a vehicle that will get me to a place of vibrant health. It will give me the ability to be active in the world and to accomplish more than I am able if I am sick or exhausted. By completing this Challenge, I will become more fully the person I was created to be, using all my gifts to make the world a better place.

I am free to eat all I want right now. No one can stop me. I can eat all the food I want right now. I don't have to stick to this Challenge. I'm not sticking to this Challenge. I can do whatever I want. No one can stop me. But I want to make positive changes. How would I feel if I gave in? I would have to start the cleanse all over. I would have to face the shame of having given in. There are good choices I can make right now, like making Maria's chocolate shake or strawberry ice cream. I am going to choose health right now. This choice will make me stronger, and each time I make this choice, the cravings will become less potent. I choose health. I choose to feel calm. Food can't make me happy.

It seems like it can and it will feel great while I eat it, but afterward, I will not feel good. I will be upset and I don't want to do that to myself. I choose to find something else to satisfy myself right now."

Feel the feeling rather than fighting the feeling. Truly, The Challenge is an amazing accomplishment and you are working hard. Remind yourself why you are doing it and remember that what you focus on will magnify. So, choose to focus on the energy and good health you are going to gain in this short amount of time. Choose to focus on how you are going to feel at the end of the ten days when you have stuck to your commitment.

Try taking a walk or going to the library and finding a good book or a stroll through the mall looking at the clothes you will fit into so soon. Do something that will completely distract you for a few hours and you will be amazed that the cravings will vanish and you will have conquered them and be stronger for it. Give yourself a pat on the back when you conquer a craving!

Remember to be looking daily at the intentions you have set for this Challenge. Cross each day off your calendar as you progress through The Challenge and consider even making a note card for hourly reference that includes your 'Why' statement and your Challenge intentions. (I'll help you with this in Chapter 3. It may also be helpful to 'construct' a space of relaxation in what Maxwell Maltz, in his book *Psycho Cybernetics*, refers to as the 'theatre of the mind." He recommends creating a space in your mind, a sanctuary that you can escape to at any moment. My space is in a cottage at a quiet and sunny, coastal retreat. Create every detail of the space in your mind. Visualize every element in the room: the décor, the color, the temperature, the smells. Make it a real place in your mind. Next, visualize the *You* you are becoming, participating in all the new activities you will engage in when your goals have been met. It's helpful to inhale an essential oil as you do this exercise and then when you find yourself wanting to go back to this special place, simply smell the oil, and you'll be right there. You might also like to download my **free 'Favorite Place Relaxation Exercise' under 'Free Downloads' at www.mariarippo.com**. Just scroll down the list until you come to it.

Rest up and stick with it. You *can* do this and you *will* be amazed at the results even after just a few days. Read back through your booklet or watch some inspiring health videos. Visit **http://www.thegreensmoothiechallenge.com/testimonials/** and watch the testimonials, knowing that you will have your own testimonial in just a few short days! What will your story be? Picture yourself telling your story. Go for a walk. Engage in something you thoroughly enjoy doing. The time will pass more quickly than you can imagine. Before you know it, you will have *done* it!

What if My Bowels are Not Moving?

It is absolutely imperative that your bowels move toxins out of your system while cleansing. One popular cleanse recommends drinking two teaspoons of Celtic salt with 32 ounces of water. I like to drink two teaspoons of salt in eight ounces of water with fresh lemon juice to make it go down and then follow this with three more glasses of water. You can also use **Smooth Move™** or **Senna tea**. Steep two teabags for 20 minutes in hot water. Drink before going to bed and then take the saltwater drink in the morning. Do it first thing, as your bowels will become very active!

Another popular method is Epsom salt. Buy a carton of Epsom salt at your local drug store and place 1 – 2 tablespoons in a glass with 8 ounces of warm water. Add the juice of ½ of a lemon and a little stevia. Drink this mixture. Make sure you have some time at home after taking this, as it too will cause your bowels to become active!

One product that really works wonders at getting at the old putrefactive matter in your colon is **Dr. Schulze's Intestinal Formula #1**. It comes in capsule form and will keep your bowels moving without causing discomfort. I have also found **Healthforce Nutritionals Intestinal Movement Formula™** to be very effective for me personally. I've also had great success with a product called **AloeMaxLax™ by Nature's Way**. My favorite new discovery that is amazing to use right along with The Challenge to totally clean out your colon is the **Blessed Herbs™ Colon Cleansing Kit™**. If you don't want to do the whole cleanse, their **Digestive Stimulator™** has worked wonders for everyone I have recommended it to. Both of these are available at **www.BlessedHerbs.com**. Again, find the option that works best for you.

If you would rather use whole foods to resolve the issue, two foods that can be helpful are fermented foods and aloe. Try making the coconut kefir and adding fresh aloe or having some fermented vegetables, such as the sauerkraut you will find in the recipe section.

Can I Drink Coffee While on The Challenge?

The Challenge is a time to give your body a rest. Coffee containing caffeine gives your adrenal glands a rush, which, in the end, robs your body of the ability to produce its own energy. It is important to take a break from this. It raises your blood pressure and prevents you from feeling fatigue that may be present, which is important to feel so you may rest. Coffee is also acidic. As you cleanse, you are bringing your pH into a more alkaline state, which is imperative for health. Most of the foods consumed in the standard American diet are acid forming. Foods such as refined sugars, processed carbohydrates and flesh foods are all acid producing. Disease thrives in an acid condition. Coffee will interrupt the process of bringing your body into an alkaline state. When you ingest acid forming foods, your body leaches minerals from itself in order to counteract the acid. Minerals are the food of the adrenals. Without minerals to nourish these all important, energy producing glands, we are left tired and in need of a caffeine boost. This adrenaline rush is actually creating the supposed need for more caffeine, which is the cause of our all too common exhaustion. Mineral deficiency is responsible for many health problems including osteoporosis.

Coffee is an irritant to the intestines. When our intestines are wounded or swollen, we do not absorb nutrients efficiently, which also robs us of vital health and energy.

Getting your java fix raises your cortisol levels as well. Cortisol is a stress hormone. When your cortisol level is high, your body will hold onto weight. Bringing this down will help you cleanse and release excess fat. Dietary stress and emotional stress also affect cortisol levels. One way to bring this down is to improve your diet to take away the dietary stress factors. Take a break from coffee for now. If you need to, have a cup of green tea instead. But, this also contains caffeine, so if you can make it without, avoiding it is the best way to give your adrenals a chance to recover.

Consider slowly weaning yourself off of coffee during the week before you begin The Challenge. You may experience a headache or even achiness during the first few days of the Challenge. Again, this is your body's cleansing reaction. It is very normal to feel less than optimal during the first few days. Consider this a sign that The Challenge is giving your body what it needs to regenerate your health! In the first few days, toxins that have been stored in fat and tissues will be dumped into your blood stream to be excreted. This process is the source of the ill feelings that follow. Welcome them, knowing that this is a sign of detoxification. It is even possible to have a fever or to break out in a rash. This is normal. Allow it to run its course.

If you release a significant amount of weight in the first few days, this is a sign that your body is retaining water which can very likely result from food allergies. As you introduce foods back into your diet, be aware of how each food makes you feel.

What Can I Drink Instead of Coffee?

Herbal teas are an important addition to your Challenge. Not only will herbal teas help tremendously with the hunger aspect, they can also aid in the detoxification process. Good herbal teas to include are chamomile, peppermint, green tea, dandelion root, ginger, milk thistle, sarsaparilla, ginseng, gotu kola, fo-ti-teng and rooibos. The one I definitely recommend drinking each day is Pau d'Arco. I have also found some satisfying herbal chai teas. Yogi™ brand has a fabulous chai tea that contains only herbs, no sweeteners. Trader Joe's has a very nice organic Ruby Red Chai as well. My favorite resource for very high quality herbal teas is **www.dragonherbs.com**. I enjoy their **Gynostemma longevity tea**. This caffeine free tea is known as an adaptogen. If you are tired, it will serve as a pick-me-up and if you are wound up, it will calm you. It has been touted as an amazing longevity herb in Chinese medicine. Some stronger herbs that I enjoy are horsetail, cats claw, nettles, holy basil and oat straw. All are very high in minerals.

Another great tea is ginger tea with fresh squeezed lemon juice. Lemon juice is cleansing for the liver and is high in Vitamin C. The liver is our main detoxification organ and we want to do all we can to support it. Ginger is an effective digestive aid as well as a metabolism booster. Combined with a bit of stevia, this is the most refreshing and cleansing tea with which to start your day. Drink this combination as you please throughout the day. You may simply prefer to have a glass of water with as much fresh lemon juice as you like. This is a simpler way to go and may seem more refreshing. Either the tea or the water is a great choice, but make sure you drink more water than tea. Water, when boiled has a different structure to it than fresh water and makes tea less hydrating. The structure of water in fruits and vegetables is perfectly matched to the needs of the human body. Listen to your body. You are ingesting a significant amount of water through the intake of greens smoothies and may not need too much other liquid. Actually, there is a point where one can take in too much liquid and dilute the electrolytes in the body. So, by all means, drink if you are thirsty, but try not to over-do it. I find that drinking a glass of water after I drink my smoothie is refreshing. The greens absorb up to three times their weight in toxic matter and I feel it is easier for the body to escort the toxins out when it is well hydrated. This may be a good idea especially if you are adding flax or chia seeds to your smoothie.

A note about herbs: Many of our modern-day medications begin as herbal concoctions. Please be mindful of the fact that herbs are strong and often times therapeutic. Some may thin your blood, decrease inflammation, decrease or increase blood pressure, etc. It is always wise to do your research and check with your health care professional before consuming herbs.

Organic Vs. Non-Organic: Is There Really a Difference?

Did you know that in the US alone, more than 1.2 billion pounds of pesticides are dumped onto our food crops on a yearly basis? Not only are pesticides toxic, the farming practices on conventional farms (those that use chemicals) are different than those practices used by organic farmers. Conventional practices include using chemicals to make plants grow and produce fruit, whereas organic farms practice amending the soil to feed it so that nutrient-dense, healthy produce can grow in it. Conventional farms amend the soil with three of the 52 necessary chemicals, phosphorous, nitrogen and potassium. That leaves the soil and resulting crops devoid of 49 necessary minerals. Many studies show that fruit and vegetables grown in organic soil contain many more nutrients than those grown in conventional methods. It seems obvious why this might be the case! Many, if not all of our diseases are associated with mineral deficiency at the core.

Another consideration is that you are trying to cleanse your body. There is already plenty of toxic buildup inside your system and adding more will, in some ways, defeat the purpose. Now if you cannot obtain organic produce, go ahead and buy conventional. According to the Environmental Working Group, the produce that is most contaminated with pesticides are apples, bell peppers, blueberries, celery, cucumbers, grapes, lettuce, nectarines, peaches, potatoes, strawberries, spinach, kale and other leafy greens, and green beans. The least contaminated produce is asparagus, cabbage cantaloupe, corn, eggplant, grapefruit, mangoes, mushrooms, onions, pineapples, plums, sweet peas, sweet potatoes, watermelon and winter squash. Romaine lettuce is found to have less contamination as well.[44] They have compiled a list of the top 12 most contaminated produce and have called it the Dirty Dozen. You can find this list and get an Android or iPhone application, as well as a printable 'take along' list for it at **www.foodnews.org**. They also have a list called the *Clean 15,* which details the produce that is the lowest in pesticides.[45]

What is the Benefit of Soaking Raw Nuts and Seeds?

In the recipe section, you will notice that some of the recipes call for soaking raw nuts and seeds. When you plant a seed in the ground, you must first water it in order for it to grow. The seed has a protective coating on it that keeps it from germinating before the proper time. This coating contains enzyme inhibitors, which basically keep the nutrients safe and largely unavailable for nourishment until the time comes for the seed to become a plant. When soaked, the enzyme inhibitors are washed away and the nutrition packed inside the seed wakes up and comes to life. The seed (or nut) begins to use up the fat for fuel. It becomes a living food, full of live enzymes and nutrients that are readily available to the one who consumes it. Soaked nuts are much more easily digested than their un-soaked counterparts.

In his book, ***Rainbow Green Live Food Cuisine***, Dr. Gabriel Cousens includes a very helpful chart that shows how long to soak each different type of nut or seed. Seeds are smaller and generally require less soaking time, such as four to six hours. Nuts on the other hand are larger and tend to require eight to twelve hours. You can visit **www.thesproutpeople.com** for a great source of sprouting seeds as well as information on soaking times. When I buy nuts and seeds, I throw all the seeds in one bowl and all the nuts in another. I add a teaspoon of sole or about a teaspoon of plain Celtic or Himalayan salt. I soak them overnight, rinse them, then put the whole batch in my dehydrator. I dehydrate them for 6 – 12 hours and then place them in Ball jars in my

---

[44] Environmental Working Group, www.ewg.org. Environmental Working Group, 2012. Web. 20 Jun 2012.
   <http://www.ewg.org/foodnews/?utm_source=201206foodnewssuba&utm_medium=email&utm_content=first-link&utm_campaign=food>.

[45] http://www.foodnews.org/walletguide.php

cupboard. This way, I eliminate the need to soak nuts too often. You can use these in trail mixes, granola, raw crackers, for grinding into flour or simply to munch on as you like. You can even flavor them before dehydrating. I like to make cinnamon toast nuts or chili lime. Just sprinkle any seasonings you like over the nuts after rinsing and before dehydrating. You can also bake them at your oven's lowest temperature. They taste just like roasted nuts, but are far more nutrient dense. You will find my favorite flavored nut recipes in Chapter 9.

What Will My Friends and Family Think?

If you stand up and be counted, from time to time you may get yourself knocked down. But remember this: A man flattened by an opponent can get up again. A man flattened by conformity stays down for good. – Thomas J. Watson, Jr.

Quite honestly, you will have friends who are your cheerleaders all the way to the finish line, and you will have friends who discourage you through the same journey. I tend to steer a little clear of, while still honoring, the ones who would like to steer me down the path that is comfortable to them, but not right for me. We cannot always expect others to agree with us. In fact, most people, such as you, who tend to reach for the stars, will face controversy. It is up to you how to handle it, but I would recommend doing so with utter love and acceptance for other people, even if you do not agree with their perspective. Others are not obligated to agree with you, and that is just fine. Do what works for you. If this is right for you and your sister or mother does not agree, allow her the right to feel that way. Don't take it personally. You are not responsible for the possible guilt or shame they feel about the way they eat and when they give you a hard time, it is really about them and these feeling that are rising in them and has nothing to do with you. Continue on your path, persevere and love those around you. Drink your smoothie with a big smile on your face and don't judge them for their choices. Before you know it, they may be asking you what is that green stuff in your martini glass. Beware: they might even want some!

What Treats Can I Have While Taking The Challenge?

An alternative to the smoothie is raw ice cream. It's another great option for those times when you feel you just *have* to eat something other than a smoothie. This is not considered "cheating." Go ahead and enjoy some of this healthy ice cream. You may also drink my "Heavenly Chocolate Milkshake" or some freshly made almond milk (recipe on page 124). Many people find that the "Hunger Eliminator" takes away any temptation to veer off of your path. You will find the recipes for all of these treats in Chapter 7. Feel free to make one of my chocolate puddings or guacamole as well. You will find these recipes in Chapter 9.

The "Heavenly Chocolate Shake" and the "Hunger Eliminator" contain some superfood ingredients. These may be unfamiliar to you so I have included an explanation of each below. Find these ingredients at The Raw Food World at **www.therawfoodworld.com**.

Are There Any Warm Alternatives to the Green Smoothie?

Raw soups as well as cooked are a great addition to your Green Smoothie Challenge. At first thought, you may be thinking that raw soup sounds cold and not so appetizing, but by raw, I mean that the soup is not heated past 115° Fahrenheit, so it can be warm and a nice alternative to the fruity, cold consistency of a smoothie. Avocado is a tasty base for a raw soup as they make it creamy. You can add corn, tomatoes, cucumbers, greens, fresh herbs, garlic, onion or anything else that sounds appetizing to you. I have included my favorite raw soup recipes in Chapter 7 as well as some additional options in Chapter 9. Also, feel free to eat cooked vegetable soup, especially if you are taking The Challenge in the winter. Just make sure to steer clear of using grains or high starch vegetables such as potatoes. You will find my Perfect Winter Challenge Broth at **www.thegreensmoothiechallenge.com.marias-blog**. Feel free to whip up some veggie soup as well. Simply start with vegetable broth and add onion, garlic, celery, carrots, parsley and some zucchini. Add seasonings such as salt, pepper and some Italian herbs. Blend and enjoy warm.

You may also consider making a simple vegetable broth. Fill a pot with water, bring it to a boil, turn down to simmer and add many chopped up vegetables. I like to add onion, garlic, potatoes, greens, celery, cabbage, turnips, carrots, beets, parsley and any others that suit you. Add a good amount of Celtic or Himalayan salt to taste. Simmer for a half hour. Strain and place in a glass jar. Store this in the refrigerator and warm up a cup of broth any time you feel like drinking it throughout the day. In the healing centers of Europe, broth is given both first thing in the morning and last thing before going to sleep. It is full of vitamins and minerals as well as being cleansing and incredibly comforting to sip. If you find you need extra protein and are not feeling well with vegetables alone, add some meat to the pot and boil until cooked. You may eat this as a soup for any meal or meals.

If you have bowel issues or constipation, consider adding flax or chia seed to your broth. Whole, organic flax or chia seeds can be added to the broth at night and left to sit in the broth until morning. This will form a gel in the broth that is healing to the lining of the stomach as well as the gut. You may warm the broth slightly before drinking. Chew the flaxseeds before swallowing.

An animal-based, but incredibly health-enhancing beverage is bone broth. So much money is spent yearly on anti-aging products. Little do people know, a simple thing such as bone broth can make an enormous difference in the appearance of the skin and can improve cellulite! Bone broth will make the skin supple. We've all seen a thin person with cellulite. It doesn't come from having excess fat; it comes from a lack of connective tissue. Collagen in the bone broth can reverse this problem because the skin will be smooth where there is sufficient connective tissue. Collagen has also been known to be healing for the lining of the intestinal tract. This will help greatly with digestive issues. Bone broth is incredibly mineral rich, meaning that it is important for your bone and teeth health. In my experience, after a few days to a week of consuming bone broth twice a day, you will see a noticeable difference in your skin and you will feel very hydrated. This is the greatest anti-aging/body transforming secret I know of and it is very inexpensive. Drink these broths anytime throughout the day during your Challenge.

How to Make Bone Broth

Fill a large stockpot ½ to ¾ full of bones of choice. Most stores sell soup bones. These are great. The most important thing is to use bones from organic, pastured, grass-fed animals. Use a variety of different bones. I make chicken broth, beef stock, fish stock, etc. Cover bones with water. Add ¼ cup of apple cider vinegar. Allow to sit for one hour. After an hour, turn stove on to medium low heat. Allow stock to come to a simmer very slowly. Once simmering, turn heat down so the broth is a continuous, but low simmer for 12–24 hours. After 12 hours, add one onion, chopped, 5 garlic cloves, 5 carrots, 5 stalks celery and a couple handfuls of any greens you have in the refrigerator.

Allow to simmer about 2–10 more hours. Add water as necessary as it will evaporate. Just don't let it get lower than the level of veggies and bones or they will burn. Once finished, strain broth into glass containers. I use ½ gallon Ball jars. I usually strain it into a big bowl first and then pour or ladle it into the jars. At this point, I add my secret ingredient. This gelatinous substance will change the appearance of your skin! It is 100% **beef gelatin** available on Amazon. I like the Bernard Jensen or Great Lakes brand. I add about ¼ cup of gelatin to each batch of broth, or you can add 1 teaspoon to 1 tablespoon to each cup of broth you drink. This is best to drink immediately upon arising and right before bed. It is incredibly hydrating and lubricating for the intestinal tract. You will see the difference! **You can also find the recipe with pictures at www.mariarippo.com**.

How Do I Get My Kids to Drink Green Smoothies?

My best advice for getting your children to drink and enjoy green smoothies is to make an extra delicious smoothie the first time. Get them into the kitchen and tell them how excited you are about a new drink you heard about. Ask if they'll help you make it. Kids love to be in the kitchen. Tell them you heard that the drinks turn into all sorts of different cool colors. Tell them you want to make one every day and see how many colors and flavors you can make. Make up fun names for them like 'Monster Juice,'

'Power Aide.' Whatever you do, at first, make fun and taste the priorities. You can add more greens once your kids have a soft spot for green smoothies.

Tell them what you've learned about the importance of enzymes and that you hadn't realized how important they were before. At the end of this book, I have included some recipes for enzyme-rich and delicious foods that most people enjoy. My neighbor kids come to my house and ask me to make many of these treats. That is the ultimate test for me to see if the food really is good!

Make the dips and the chocolate shake. Always introduce kids to healthy food by making the most delicious recipes you can find. This will open their minds and help them feel excited about the new options. Often people are just convinced that healthy food tastes bad. Surprise them!

It is important to implement new foods slowly so that your children do not feel it is a chore to eat them. They love finger foods, so veggie sticks, raw crackers and dips are a great place to start. Most kids enjoy sweet foods too, so make sure you start out with sweet green smoothies. Let them decide what to put in each day. Educate them about why green is good. If you are excited, there will be a better chance they will be excited. If you involve them and allow them to get into the kitchen and be creative, how can they not be excited too? If you are tentative or afraid they won't like them, they will pick up on that and you will be right, so focus instead on the time together and the creative fun you will have. Laugh if it tastes bad and feed it to the worms in your garden. Serve green smoothies in a special glass. Make it a celebration! See Chapter 7 for my tasty "Kid Approved Smoothie," the "Slurpy Smoothie" or "Robin's Creamsicle," as well as tasty options from other moms who have mastered the art of getting children to beg for smoothies.

Unfamiliar Ingredients

In this section, I will explain some possibly unfamiliar foods you will find throughout my recipes. You can find most of them online through The Raw Food World at **www.therawfoodworld.com**.

Celtic and Himalayan Salt – What are They and Why are They Recommended?

In order to collect Celtic salt, pure seawater is transferred through a series of evaporation ponds. A hot, dry climate allows the evaporation process to occur naturally, leaving behind only pure salt crystals, naturally rich in valuable trace minerals, which are not present in regular salt. These salts actually add essential nutrients to your diet, while

---

[46] www.cultureoflifeshoppe.com

refined salts are harmful to your health. You can use them as you would table salt. They will enhance the flavors of all the beautiful foods you make.

Himalayan salt comes from the foothills of the Himalayan Mountains in Pakistan. This is referred to as "white gold" and contains all 84 elements found in your body. It is completely unprocessed. Your body can utilize this salt in ways that does not cause water retention. It actually assists with the body's processes of elimination. The salt is mined as very large crystals that are simply ground down into salt with no processing.

This type of salt has nothing in common with table salt. They are not even in the same category. Your table salt is actually 97.5% sodium chloride and 2.5% chemicals such as moisture absorbents and iodine. Dried at over 1,200° Fahrenheit, the excessive heat alters the natural chemical structure of the salt. Many natural health practitioners strongly advise to stay far away from regular table salt. In fact, it is called one of the 'four white devils which are white flour, white sugar, table salt and pasteurized dairy.

Sole (Pronounced Soul-ay)

Sole is an inexpensive way to get a large amount of essential minerals into your system. Before you begin The Challenge, make a batch of sole so you can add a teaspoon to a glass of lemon water or fresh green juice each day. This will greatly increase the amount of minerals you are taking in. To make the sole, drop a pure **Himalayan salt crystal** into a glass jar filled with water (use a plastic lid). I prefer a jar that holds about three cups of water. Let it sit overnight. When you notice that the salt is dissolved, add another crystal and continue to do so until the crystals will no longer dissolve. You can expect to use two or three crystals. When you notice that the crystal does not dissolve, the water is at full saturation and the sole is ready for use. Simply take a teaspoon of sole and add it to each smoothie. As an alternative, you may add it to your morning water with a squeeze of fresh lemon juice and a dash of stevia. You will want to use pure Himalayan salt crystals to make this recipe. This will help to give you energy and hydration.

What is Raw Cacao? Is it Chocolate?

Chocolate comes from the cacao bean. When in its raw form it is referred to as "cacao" and when roasted and processed it is commonly known as "cocoa." This is the most revered food of the rainforest. It has been known from ancient times as the "food of the gods." According to nutritionist and raw-food guru, David Wolfe, raw cacao is the highest natural source of magnesium, chromium, iron *and* antioxidants. It is thirty times higher in antioxidants than red wine and twenty times higher than green tea. It has

---

[47] http://products.mercola.com/himalayan-salt/

much higher antioxidant levels than acai. I occasionally have my antioxidant level tested, and after I began eating raw cacao daily, my antioxidant levels shot through the roof! I no longer eat it daily because it's a bit too stimulating for me, but I love to have it as a treat. A word of caution: if your adrenals are not strong, you might use carob instead, as it is not stimulating. Remember, less can sometimes be more.

What is Lecithin?

Another popular name for this amazing product is "let's be thin." OK, that's probably all you need to hear, but just in case you'd like to know more about this ingredient, I thought I'd share why it's good for your health. Lecithin is an emulsifier that allows fat and water to mix. This enables the body to break down fats and eliminate them rather than storing them. It supports healthy triglyceride and cholesterol levels. It is a potent source of choline and inositol. Choline is important for healthy liver function and plays a key role in neurotransmitter function. A deficiency in it can lead to fat buildup in and around the liver as well as nerve degeneration, senile dementia, high blood cholesterol and liver cancer. It is also a thickening agent, which adds a creamy texture to milkshakes, especially if you let it sit for ten minutes before you drink it. Healthforce Nutritionals is the only brand I recommend, as it is non-GMO (not a genetically modified organism). If you use a different brand, just make sure it says "Non-GMO" because most soy is genetically modified. I like to eat my food in its natural form, not in a form that has been altered by man.

What are Tocotrienols?

Tocotrienols are a newly discovered, pure form of vitamin E and a good source of the B vitamins. The experts claim that tocotrienols are 40 to 60 times more potent than the more well known form of vitamin E, tocopherols. Tocotrienols are a class of the tocopherols that were unknown until recently. At present time, there are four named tocotrienols which are alpha, beta, gamma and delta. Symptoms of a vitamin E deficiency include **acne**, anemia, Lou Gehrig's disease, muscular dystrophy, gallstones, certain cancers, Parkinson's and Alzheimer's diseases. Sufficient levels of vitamin E can protect against heart disease, viral infections, cancer, strokes and fibrocystic breast disease. Gabriel Cousens, MD, recommends taking 1–2 tablespoons of this nutrient per day. So why not get it in the form of a tantalizing chocolate beverage?

---

[48] Wolfe, David, *Superfoods,* North Atlantic Books, Berkeley, CA 2009.

[49] Shazzie, *Evie's Kitchen: Raising an Ecstatic Child,* Rawcreation Ltd., 2008.

[50] http://www.cultureoflifestore.com/p408/Tocotrienols,+16oz,+Sunfood+Nutrition/ product_info.html

What is Mucuna Pruriens?

Mucuna is known as a popular coffee substitute. It is a bean that grows on a climbing vine. It is most notably used in Ayurvedic medicine for sexual diseases and nervous disorders.

The seeds of mucuna pruriens contain a large amount of a substance known as L-Dopa. This substance is a precursor to dopamine in the brain. While it is not dopamine, it is an amino acid that converts to dopamine once ingested. It is the most potent natural source of L-dopa known. Upon ingestion, it immediately nourishes the dopamine neurotransmitter pathway.

A dopamine deficiency can be responsible for depression, cravings, addictive tendencies, low libido, fatigue, weight gain, muscle tenseness and trembling, as in the case of Parkinson's disease. In fact, mucuna pruriens is a traditional Ayurvedic remedy for Parkinson's disease. An anecdotal testimony tells about an experience with a woman who was trembling with Parkinson's and when given a **dose** of mucuna pruriens her trembling immediately ceased.

This legume is known to help improve the following: sleep, body fat, appearance of cellulite, skin, bone density, libido, lean muscle mass, blood **sugar levels**, mood, fatigue, depression, immunity and cholesterol. It is also known to give strength to the heart, kidneys, liver and **lungs**. Mucuna is sold in powder form as a simple addition to juice or a smoothie. It is recommended to mix 15 grams of the powder with juice.

What is Yacon Powder?

The yacon plant produces tuberous roots that are edible and quite sweet. This is a beneficial addition to your diet because the tubers contain an element called fructooligosacharides (FOS). These promote colon health because they are the perfect food for the good bacteria that reside there. This enables the good bacteria to flourish to promote a balanced colon ecology that is necessary for optimal wellness. The tuberous roots of the yacon plant contain the most FOS of any plant in the world.

Yacon powder is a great sweetener because of its sweetness but also because the FOS, which creates the sweet taste, is not digestible by the body. It never enters the bloodstream as sugar. This makes yacon suitable for diabetics as well as those who are attempting to shed unwanted pounds.

---

[51] Wolfe, David, Interviews. I have learned these facts over the years by listening to David Wolfe.

[52] http://herbal-powers.com/macunapruriens1.html

54

The yacon root is high in antioxidants, and studies suggest that it assists the body in the absorption of calcium. Look for it in powder, syrup or dried fruit form.

What are Chia Seeds?

Chia seeds are a highly nutrient-dense food. You probably know of them from the funny Chia Pets you see in stores. Yes, these are the same type of seed, but the ones used to make Chia Pets do not have the same nutritional value. I like to think of this food as one of God's gifts to the waistline! Besides being incredibly nutritious, they can keep you feeling full for hours. Chia seeds contain five times more calcium than milk and conveniently contain boron, which helps to transfer that calcium into your bones. They have twice as much protein as any other seed or grain. They also contain all the amino acids making them a complete protein. They are high in Omega 3 essential fatty acids (EFAs), which is important because the Standard American Diet (SAD) is overly high in Omega 6 EFAs and not high enough in the Omega 3 fatty acids. Boosting these particular EFAs can have an enormously positive effect on your health. Your body cannot produce these oils and they are an essential part of a healthy diet. Our bodies must have these EFAs for normal cell functioning. They promote heart health and brain function. My favorite part about chia seeds is they become gelatinous when you hydrate them. They are a perfect thickening agent for puddings and shakes. I thoroughly enjoy both and they fill me up for hours! When using ground chia seeds, it's important to use freshly ground seeds. You can use a coffee mill for this job. You may also add them to your smoothie before blending and they will be ground in the process of blending the smoothie. Grinding the seeds allows the nutrients to become available to the body for use.

Chia seeds help to control blood sugar levels making them a diabetic-friendly food and a perfect addition to smoothies. Their soluble fiber causes carbohydrates to be slowly released into the body. This also offers an appetite suppressing affect, helping you to feel full for an extended time without taking in extra calories. You'll find my "Chocolate Chia Pudding" in the recipe section in Chapter 9. Feel free to eat this while on The Challenge instead of adding the seeds to your smoothie. Some people feel dehydrated when they eat chia in this manner daily, so make sure to drink plenty of water if you choose to consume these seeds. An alternative is to make a hydrating chia gel that you can simply add to your smoothie.

For extra hydration and a soothing drink for the intestinal lining, you can make a gel from chia seeds and drink it daily. Simply combine ⅓ cups whole chia seeds with 2 cups water and allow to sit overnight. Store this in your refrigerator and drink a small amount of the gel throughout the day. This gel will last about one week in your refrigerator.

---

[53] Wolfe, David, *Superfoods,* North Atlantic Books, Berkeley, CA 2009

What are Flax Seeds?

Flax seeds are the highest plant sources of Omega 3 EFAs making them a recommended heart healthy food by the American Heart Association. They, like chia seeds, are very high in Omega 3 EFAs and very low in Omega 6 EFAs. We tend to throw off the balance of these essential nutrients because we consume so many Omega 6 fatty acids in our diets and tend not to consume much Omega 3. For this reason, it is recommended that we supplement with Omega 3 rich foods. Flax and chia are the highest plant-based sources of Omega 3 fatty acids readily available, although Sacha Inchi oil is proving to be a higher source, but harder to come by. Flaxseeds are the richest plant source of lignans. Lignans are phytonutrients found in foods containing high amounts of dietary fiber. Lignans are known to be anti-viral, anti-fungal and anti-bacterial in nature. One study found that men whose diets were high in lignans had a significantly lower risk of dying from coronary heart disease or cardiovascular disease than those whose diets were low in lignans Flax seeds are full of the all-important plant fiber. This makes flax an excellent way to control blood sugar levels. Flax seeds absorb toxins and enable the body to excrete them by keeping the bowels regular. They are anti-inflammatory and have been known to relieve pain associated with inflammation.

The best way to use flax is to freshly grind the seeds using a coffee grinder and then add them to a smoothie. Only use freshly ground flaxseeds as they lose their oils quickly and become rancid after being ground. I have found one exception to this. Omega Nutrition has a special process for grinding their **flax seeds** which allows them to be shelf stable for one year. The company has tested their seeds for rancidity and has found that there is no change after one year. I trust this company and use their ground flax seeds myself. If you use them whole, it is best to soak them first in pure water for an hour or so before using.

What is Coconut Oil and is it REALLY Healthy?

Coconut oil is believed by some to be the healthiest oil for us to consume. In Sanskrit (the language of ancient India), the coconut palm is known as kalpa vriksha, meaning "the tree that supplies all that is needed to live." It is heat stable, meaning that the nutritive benefits stay intact when the oil is heated above a certain temperature. It is thermogenic, helping to improve the metabolism. It is a heart healthy and slimming fat.

---

[54] Thompson LU. Experimental studies on lignans and cancer. Baillieres Clin Endocrinol Metab. 1998;12(4):691-705. (PubMed)

[55] Vanharanta M, Voutilainen S, Rissanen TH, Adlercreutz H, Salonen JT. Risk of cardiovascular disease-related and all-cause death according to serum concentrations of enterolactone: Kuopio Ischaemic Heart Disease Risk Factor Study. Arch Intern Med. 2003;163(9):1099-1104. (PubMed)

[56] Wolfe, David, *Superfoods*. North Atlantic Books, Berkeley, CA 2009

[57] Calbom, Cherrie, *The Juice Lady's Turbo Diet*. Siloam, A Strang Company, Lake Mary, FL, 2010.

Your body does not store the fat from coconut oil. Instead, it converts it to fuel, making it a food that provides energy. Coconut oil does have the ability to raise cholesterol levels, so it is good for those with low cholesterol; but if yours is high, you may want to be careful with this ingredient. Coconut oil is high in lauric acid, making this healing oil well known for its antifungal, antibacterial and antiviral properties. For this reason, it is often used to improve intestinal health. I prefer to use Omega Nutrition's organic, virgin coconut oil.

What is Stevia?

Stevia is a plant native to western North America as well as South America. It is mostly grown for it's sweet leaves for use as a natural sweetener. Stevia is about three hundred times sweeter than sugar. A little goes a long way. There are different forms of stevia and I will explain each so you can choose the one that best fits your needs. The stevia plant produces green leaves so the purest form of stevia is green. It is simply ground stevia leaves. It can tend to have a bitter aftertaste, but if you use just enough, it can add a very sweet flavor. My favorite form of stevia is the **SweetLeaf™** whole leaf stevia extract liquid. It is a dark liquid made with minimal processing and is a perfect, natural addition to green smoothies. The next form is the white powder. This is refined through a water extraction process and my favorite brand is **SweetLeaf™**. Stevia often comes with a tiny scooper so my recipes call for 5 scoops of stevia, which is the amount I have found to add the perfect sweetness without the bitter aftertaste. Five scoops are equal to ⅛ teaspoon. You may need to adjust the amount to fit your unique taste for stevia. You can also add this sweetener to your teas or other beverages in place of artificial sweeteners or sugar. It's the perfect natural alternative. SweetLeaf™ brand also offers liquid stevia with added flavor such as vanilla, chocolate, raspberry, English toffee, grape, etc. If you find other brands at your local store, make sure there is no added sugar or other ingredients. It should state "pure stevia extract" as the only ingredient.

What is Ashwagandha?

Ashwagandha is an adaptogenic herb that's known for helping the body adapt to stress. It is used in Ayurvedic medicine to treat hypertension and stress-related illnesses. It is known to be supportive to the nervous system, to give energy and vitality and to increase libido. I like to say it gives you back your libido for life!

What is Xylitol?

Xylitol is a sugar substitute known to be safe for diabetics, as it does not affect insulin levels. Xylitol is a sugar alcohol and is recommended for use by people who need to stay away from sugar. I only recommend using the pure birch xylitol. Two good brands are the **Ultimate Sweetener™** and **Smartsweet™**.

What is Rapadura?

Rapadura is organic sugar in its purest form. It is an unrefined sweetener that looks like ground up sugar cane. Rapadura is also called 'whole cane sugar'. Because it is not refined like other sugars, it retains most of its essential nutrients, vitamins and minerals. Refined sugar is damaging to the body because the naturally occurring minerals have been removed during the refining process. In order for the sugar to be digested, minerals are required. Once the minerals have been removed, the body must 'borrow' minerals from the teeth and bones to digest the sugar, which is one reason sugar can be so damaging to the body. With all its minerals intact, Rapadura has a unique caramel-like flavor and is my favorite sweetener for baking and sweetening food and drinks. I use the Rapunzel brand whole cane sugar (formerly known as Rapadura).

What is Raw Honey?

Pure, unfiltered, unpasteurized raw honey is one of the most healing foods on the planet. It is packed with live enzymes, vitamins, minerals and antioxidants. Raw honey has been shown to inhibit the growth of pathogens in food and food spoilage organisms. Scientists at Cornell University, Geneva, New York report 'Honey has been used as a topical and gastrointestinal remedy for thousands of years, and has recently gained recognition from the medical field. The growth of many microorganisms associated with disease or infection is inhibited by honey.' I have used honey to heal wounds and it works better than any other remedy you can buy.

---

[58] www.honeygardens.com, *Honey Education*. Extracted February 19, 2012.

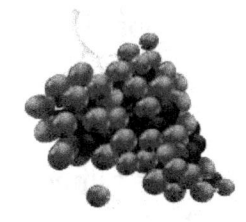

CHAPTER 3
Getting Prepared

Defining Your Why

Now that you are fully convinced that this is a Challenge you are ready to take on, it is time to consider "why" you are going to do something so crazy! This is a time to dig a little deeper than simply taking The Challenge to release weight or to have more energy. Sit down and really think about *why* you want to release weight or *why* you would like to have more energy. Do you have a family? Maybe you'd like to be around to see your grandchildren grow up and have enough energy to chase them around. Maybe you want to make sure you are healthy enough to provide for your family. Be sure to use positive words for your reasons such as "I am, I have, I will, I choose" instead of using negative verbiage such as "I can't, I won't, I don't." For example, you might say, "I am going to take The Challenge because I don't have any energy." Instead, say, "I am going to take The Challenge to increase my energy level." Speak to yourself in a positive tone. Go deep into defining your reasons why. Even ask yourself: "Why do I want to provide for my family, have more energy or be around to play with my grandchildren?" Keep asking why until you have it really nailed down. Imagine, vividly, what your life will look like once you have released weight or gained energy. What will be new and different about your life? What are some things that will change? What will you be able to do that you are currently unable do? Create a detailed movie in your mind of what you will do when you are thinner and full of vitality. What will you do with the extra time you have as a result of needing less sleep? Think of all the positive ways these changes will affect your life and write them down. Even create a vision board with pictures or a video, called a mind movie, so you can be reminded, in pictures, daily, about your goals. When you feed your subconscious mind in this way, it will lead you right to the necessary tools to fulfill your intentions.

You may want to take The Challenge in order to get on track with your eating. Maybe you are feeling undisciplined in this area, and you need an extra boost of motivation to start eating more healthfully. You are free to make all of your own decisions. It is so easy to get into a rut of making less-than-optimal decisions around food. We are constantly bombarded with unhealthy options to choose from. Now is the time to realize that the choice is *always* yours. You are in total control of what goes into your mouth. If you do tend to make unhealthy choices, know that you are absolutely normal because many of us struggle here as well. You may even feel obsessed and compulsive at times. You might feel like I have felt so often, that it feels impossible to think of anything but food. This is simply a habit or a way to escape from the stresses of day-to-day life. It is said that it takes three weeks to break a habit. Let this be the beginning of new choices for yourself. Decide right now that you are going to give your energy to more productive things, rather than giving in to unhealthy eating choices. Focus on the health you are bringing into your life, rather than what you are *not* eating.

You may also desire to implement a good exercise routine. Now is a great time to do this as you will have more time to exercise because you are spending less time eating. Maybe your goal is to release some extra weight so that exercising is not such a chore for you. Whatever it is that will motivate you during times of intense hunger, write this down and refer back to it daily. This must be a 'why' that really matters to you. Take a few minutes here to contemplate and write down 'why' you are going to take this Challenge. If you are having a hard time figuring out your 'why', try the following exercise, which I learned from Oriah Mountain Dreamer. Say you want to release twenty-five pounds. You would then write the following: "It doesn't matter to me if I release twenty five pounds, what I really want is _____". Continue with this exercise until you really figure out what it is you want in life. What will you have after you have released this weight that you do not have now? What is missing in your life that you truly desire? What is your deep longing? What do you daydream about being different in your life?

Figuring out why you are doing something may seem like a large task. Here are some ideas you might consider focusing on as you decide what your major motivation is for taking this Challenge. Close your eyes for a minute and visualize what changes will take place as a result of taking The Challenge.

- What is your desired outcome?
- Will you have more energy?
- Will you fit into your clothes more easily?
- Will you be thrilled when you look in the mirror?
- Will you be able to chase your children or grandchildren?
- Will you experience peace? Will your acid reflux disappear?
- Will your food cravings vanish?
- Will your food obsessions stop nagging you?

- Will you need less sleep?

- Will you have more clear, mental focus?

- Will you have more trust for yourself?

- What will be different when your Challenge is complete?

- What outcomes do you most desire to experience?

- What are you unable to do right now, that you will be able to do when you are healthier and lighter?

See your life changing in these ways. Allow these changes to become a reality in your mind. What does it feel like to be in that place you desire to be, to fulfill the intentions you choose for yourself to achieve and to wake up each morning in this new body with these new outcomes? Be this new person in your mind for a few minutes. Experience the new you and now write down the three new changes that you desire the most. Write them all down if you wish! This is your 'Why' statement.

_____

_____

_____

_____

_____

_____

_____

_____

_____

_____

_____

_____

_____

Once you are clear on your 'why', the next step is to draw a picture of your future self, five years from now. Draw this future self, bowing in gratitude to your current self for taking the important steps you are about to take so you can get where you want to be. Make sure that you convey the new changes in the future self, as they have already happened. You may also choose to write a letter from your future self, five or ten years from now, thanking you for doing the hard work of making these changes. Get as detailed as you can.

I find that for me personally, weight loss is not enough of a motivation for me to stick to the Challenge. Watching my weight drop certainly will motivate me as I step on the scale each day, if I choose to do so, but in times of intense hunger or cravings, it is the things I hold much more dearly than the number on that scale, that keep me on track. My number one motivator is high energy. I tend to naturally have a lower energy level. I like to accomplish a lot every day and I want to have the energy to do that. I want to be able to stay up at night with my family, helping with homework, reading to my girls or talking over tea with my husband. If I get too tired, I am not in a good mood at night and my family doesn't get the best of me. I also like to wake up in the quiet, early hours of the morning to read, meditate, chant or exercise before the sun peaks it face out from behind the night sky. Another big motivator for me is clear skin and bright whites of my eyes. I do not have these things unless I eat very healthy. In fact, when I don't eat healthy I become moody, hormonal and monster-like. I don't want to be that way, so choosing to eat unhealthy food for me leaves a lot of choices on the table. Usually I find it is just not worth it! But, if it all came down to a number on a scale, most of the time I myself might choose to eat more than I need to or choose to eat things that I know are not optimal. I just don't want the other outcomes those choices give me and that's what keeps me on track in times of temptation. It is conscious thought about my choices and the resulting outcome. What motivates you? What changes do you want to see more than you want to eat things that will keep you right where you are? And what do you need to shed other than weight? Negative beliefs? Resentment? What is no longer serving you? Are you ready to let it go?

> *"People with goals succeed because they know where they are going... It's as simple as that."* — *Earl Nightingale*

> *"There is one quality that one must possess to win, and that is definiteness of purpose, the knowledge of what one wants, and a burning desire to possess it."* — *Napoleon Hill*

I'd like to note that not all people set and achieve goals in the same way. If you are one to set a goal and attain it, great, you found what works for you. If you are one to set a goal and then sabotage it and end up achieving frustration instead, then I would suggest using visualization of where you want to be instead of writing out specific goals. Focus on your 'why' and the how will show up for you. Be very patient and compassionate with yourself as you find what does and what does not work for you. If one method does not work for you, it not because you are somehow flawed and a failure; it is simply that that particular method is not what works for your personality. Self-sabotage can actually be a beautiful gift when we are open to it, instead of resisting it. When we become curious about it and notice the thoughts we have after the sabotaging behavior takes place, we have the golden key to unlock the door of what is holding us back. This usually involves working with a coach or therapist, and is the work I do for myself and with my own clients.

I invite you to take some time and write down why you are going to take this Challenge.

_____

_____

_____

_____

_____

_____

_____

_____

_____

_____

_____

_____

_____

_____

Now that you have your 'why' statement complete, you are ready to get going. You may choose to start The Challenge slowly by easing into it. That is a good idea for some people. I tend to want to jump right in when I feel the desire to cleanse. Do what works best for you.

Releasing Weight

Be prepared to release a good amount of weight for the first few days. After this, it will most likely taper off a bit and continue more slowly. There may be some days where you release no weight. Other days you lose one-quarter pound and then all of a sudden you will lose two pounds. This is very normal. Know that your body is hard at work and happy. It is burning fat for fuel and releasing toxins, and healing. There is so much more to this than purely weight loss. One temptation may be to obsess over what the scale says. If this happens, putting your scale away for a time or forever would be a good option. You may even like to measure your waist or experience your clothing becoming looser instead of stepping on the scale, as this may be a more reliable way to watch the physical changes unfold. In my experience, weighing in works for a small number of people, but when our focus is on the scale, it takes us outside of our body. When we rely on feedback from sources outside ourselves, we cease to listen to our body. It is imperative to come into a supportive relationship with our body. I invite you to find a goal that is much more meaningful to you than simply weight loss. What does the weight loss mean to you?

What you focus on always magnifies. If you choose to focus on what you are not eating, most likely you will have a difficult time thinking of much other than these foods and you'll really crave them. But, if you choose to focus on the health benefits of taking The Challenge, you'll be more likely to stay motivated to work towards your goals. Focus on how your clothes are fitting and the extra energy you have. Focus on the good nutrition you are adding to your body and the toxins you are releasing. Focus on how you are going to look and feel, after the ten days are over.

Everyone is different, and your rate of weight loss may be slower than you had hoped. Some people experience a large amount of weight loss right away only to become discouraged in the next few days when the scale does not show that they are releasing. Most often, your clothes are still becoming looser. Your body is adjusting to some big changes so do not allow the scale to discourage you. Get excited about fitting into that pair of jeans you haven't been able to wear for a long time.

Make sure you are drinking *a lot* of pure water. Hydration is key for weight loss as well as detoxification. It speeds up the fat loss process too.

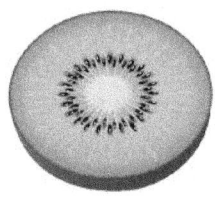

CHAPTER 4
Customizing Your Challenge

The Green Smoothie Challenge is about being kind to your body. It is not a perfection contest. It is not about deprivation and starvation. It is not even really about releasing excess weight, although most people do release a significant amount. The Green Smoothie Challenge is about nourishing your body, refreshing your soul, reviving your spirit. It's about clearing your mind and giving your body a much needed break from digesting foods it was never meant to ingest (Can you say soda, fast-food and processed carbohydrates?) It is about taking a break from the all too common food obsessions many of us struggle with so you can reassess your relationship with food. It's about becoming energized on a new level. It's about new beginnings, getting back on track and creating balance in your life. Releasing weight is just an added benefit!

The following information will help you understand the options you have for taking The Challenge. Simply choose the one that will work best for you in your current situation. The first option may be too big of a jump for you at first. If you fit into this common category, congratulate yourself for being honest and truthful. A 10-day Green Smoothie Challenge is a big deal and not meant as torture for anyone! If you prefer to take smaller steps towards health or if you have taken many medications in your life and your diet has consisted of much processed food and commercially raised animal products, The Challenge may bring about detoxification too quickly. In this case, choose one of the other versions to follow. All of these additional options are still very cleansing and offer more calories and slower detoxification. As I have said previously, there is not one method or diet that works for every person. Doing a modified version is still a Challenge and you can be very proud of your accomplishments when you have completed any step that brings you closer to attaining your health goals! I even modify the Challenge myself and I am the creator of it!

Keep your particular personality in mind as you choose your Challenge. Some people do great sticking to their commitments; they thrive on it. Others struggle greatly with the mind games that are common when abstaining from particular foods. Still others almost automatically want to go against what they set out to do before taking their first step (ahem, that would be me). That's OK. It's not right or wrong. It just *is*. If this is you, accept that it *is* and choose the option that does not involve being too strict. This is a good place to start and then, if you like, you can work towards the other versions as you feel comfortable doing so. The most important thing is not to set yourself up for failure. If you choose one option and end up not sticking to it, simply take that as feedback that another option might work more effectively for your personality and place in life. Be kind and patient with yourself. You have not failed; you have simply discovered the option that does not best suit you right now. It's OK! You are one step closer to discovering YOUR Challenge!! In fact, how can you find what does work for you until you experience what does not? The most important thing is to honor yourself right where you are and start there.

Remember that food is comforting. Eating when we are stressed out, sad, angry or frustrated is in fact, calming. It is actually a form of escape from feeling your emotions. It is a way to *not* deal with them. It is also very common in today's world. If this describes you, own it, and love and accept yourself anyway. Resisting it only causes it to persist. It is absolutely not something you need to hide. Eating *does* feel good. It is, after-all, one of life's greatest pleasures. Becoming aware of it is half the battle won. The other half is learning to feel those emotions instead of numbing them with food and learning how to effectively let them go. If this is you I highly recommend reading **Eating in the Light of the Moon** by Dr. Anita Johnston. You can listen to my **radio interview with her at www.blogtalkradio.com/enlightenmeradio** for amazing tools to overcome emotional eating. I also recommend reading **The End of Overeating**, by David A. Kessler, MD. Feel free to switch between Challenges too. If you are like me, sometimes you need to experience something before you can tell if it's right for you. Again, take the outcome as feedback, not failure. It's actually important to experience how we don't want to live before we can learn how we do want to live.

> *Our greatest glory is not in never falling but in rising every time we fall. – Confucius*

Please remember that it is imperative to speak to your physician before making drastic changes to your diet.

The following pages contain The Challenge options for you to choose from, including The Original Challenge, The Original Challenge with a Bit More Crunch, The Intermediate Challenge, The Get Your Feet Wet Challenge, The Performance Enhancer and Tips for Pregnant and Nursing Moms.

The Original Challenge

The original version of The Green Smoothie Challenge is the original cleanse that has helped many people release large amounts of weight in a short amount of time. It is energizing, mind clearing and mood enhancing. It is a Challenge for people who choose to cleanse more rapidly and are willing to take a more extreme approach. It is the simplest version as far as food preparation and possibly the most complex as far as the mental discipline of staying away from most food. Some people do best when abstaining from chewing food altogether for the ten days. Others prefer to munch all day long on fresh, organic fruits and vegetables. The choice is all yours. The key is in finding what *does* work for you. This is not meant to be about self-deprivation, but instead, about rejuvenation of the mind, body and spirit and about taking a break from the damaging foods many people ingest on a daily basis.

You will find a grocery list in Chapter 6 that corresponds to the first ten smoothie recipes in Chapter 7. These original recipes allowed my husband to release fifteen pounds in nine days. They are the same recipes that many people whose testimonials you have read, also followed.

Tips for Taking Any Version of The Challenge.

Upon arising, drink a glass or two of water with the juice of ½ a lemon and a pinch of **Celtic or Himalayan** salt. I also like to take my greens in the morning with lemon juice. It's the first thing that goes into my body every day! Lemon is cleansing and hydrating. A pinch of good salt allows the cells to absorb water more easily. Use only a small pinch. I also like to add two drops of **Young Living essential oil** because this is the oil from the lemon peel. It is known to have anti-cancer and liver cleansing properties. Find the oil at **www.transformationaloils.marketingscents.com**.

Make your smoothies for the day so everything is prepared and easily accessible when hunger strikes. Each Green Smoothie Challenge smoothie recipe at the beginning of Chapter 7 is enough for an entire day. Instead of having variety each day, I recommend drinking the same smoothie all day and trying a new recipe each day. This will save a lot of time. Pour your smoothie into one large jug or use four separate jars, one for each smoothie serving.

After preparing your smoothie, drink your first portion, sipping it slowly and even chewing it a bit before swallowing. This will mix the smoothie in with your digestive juices for maximum nutrient absorption.

Feel free to follow each smoothie with some water. It is wise to drink spring water, reverse osmosis or filtered water. Most health food stores have water purification systems that allow you to fill your own water bottles for an affordable price.

In between smoothies, you are free to munch on fresh fruit and vegetables. Just pack up a variety to take with you at the beginning of the day. Some of my favorites are carrots, celery, jicama, avocado, red bell peppers, cucumbers, tomatoes, apples, berries, pears, grapes, grapefruit, kiwi and oranges. A favorite snack of many Challengers is my guacamole with fresh cut veggies to dip in it. I love to use jicama, carrots and celery as the 'chips' for this filling treat. Celery is naturally salty and the jicama can be sliced in the shape of chips. You will find my super fabulous guacamole recipe in Chapter 9. This is a very welcome treat during the height of your afternoon hunger. I do not recommend using avocado in your smoothie if you are going to have this as a snack unless releasing weight is not a goal for you.

At dinnertime, you may wish to have a big plate of steamed vegetables. I find that if you have a family who is eating dinner, getting through that time of day can be very challenging. My husband and I discovered that if we simply steamed some broccoli and seasoned it with some herbs such as **Herbamare®** or **Braggs® Organic Sprinkle**, we had a much easier time cleansing through the evening hours. Another option is to sauté some onion and garlic in coconut oil and add some chopped, dark leafy greens such as kale, collards, chard or any of your choosing. Sauté for about five minutes, stirring occasionally. Add some **raw apple cider vinegar** and seasoning or **Celtic**, **Himalayan** or **Real™** salt for a delicious treat. You might even like to try this recipe using zucchini and tomatoes instead of leafy greens, leaving out the vinegar. The evening is also a good time to sprinkle some cinnamon in your tea. This treat will warm your tummy as well as help reduce your appetite.

Choose three more times during the day to consume your smoothies. There is not a particular time you need to do this, just listen to your hunger and try not to let it get too intense before drinking some more smoothie. If your hunger does get very intense, remind yourself that it is not as urgent as it feels, unless you are diabetic or hypoglycemic in which case you might talk to your doctor about how to go about taking The Challenge. Hunger will actually get very extreme and then it will suddenly disappear almost as if your body decided that it asked eagerly enough and now it is going to go about some other work. I like to make it a game of "let's see how long it takes before this hunger goes away." It's actually an interesting experiment to do. Relaxing through it seems to bring strength and confidence. I tell my kids when they get really hungry, "Just breathe, it's really going to be OK. It is just your body asking for nourishment. That's it. It is not as urgent as it feels and if you relax through it, you will actually stop feeling hungry!" This is a good time to breathe deeply and relax through it.

Another welcome addition to The Challenge is vegetable soup. Find the **cleansing veggie soup** recipe at **www.thegreensmoothiechallenge.com/recipes**.

The Original Challenge

Your day on The Original Challenge may look like this:

6 am: Arise and drink two glasses of water with a pinch of salt and fresh squeezed lemon juice along with two drops of lemon essential oil, optional (optional, take green powder.)

7 am: Drink your first portion of smoothie, about 16 ounces, followed by a glass of water, if desired.

8 am: Drink a cup of green tea, herbal tea or broth.

10 am: Drink your second portion of smoothies, again, about 16 ounces, followed by a glass of water, if desired.

11:30 am: Eat an apple or other fruit or some veggie sticks.

1 pm: Drink your third portion of green smoothie.

3 pm: Snack on guacamole with veggie 'chips' or Maria's Heavenly Chocolate Shake. You will find this recipe in Chapter 7, as well as Chapter 9.

5 pm: Have some steamed vegetables or one of my warm, raw soups or cleansing vegetable soup found in Chapter 7 or 9.

7 pm: Drink your last portion of green smoothie or have some strawberry ice cream. Try adding different fruits to it as well. My family loves peach ice cream!

9 pm: Drink some dandelion tea, pau d'arco or any tea or broth of your choosing. Add cinnamon to your tea, if desired. Another great bedtime tea is Senna. You can buy bulk Senna herb at your local health food store. Another option is **Smooth Move Tea™**. It will help you to have a good elimination the following morning. Simply steep one or two teabags for 20 minutes before enjoying. Feel free to add **stevia powder** or liquid to your tea. My preferred brand is **SweetLeaf™ Pure Stevia Whole Leaf Concentrate liquid**. This liquid is dark, as opposed to the processed liquids, which are clear. The darkness is a result of it being preserved in its natural state. Stevia comes from a green leaf.

9:30 pm: Go to bed and get some good rest. Rest is essential for good health. Go to bed even earlier if you are able and especially if you feel tired. Listen to your body!

The Original Challenge with a Bit More Crunch

In addition to drinking smoothies and munching on fresh fruit and veggies throughout the day, have an avocado with fresh lemon juice, Celtic salt and cayenne pepper. Eat a big green salad with a large variety of colorful veggies and one of my dressings for lunch and dinner. You will find my dressing recipes in the recipe section. You may also snack on raw (preferably soaked) nuts and seeds such as almonds, sunflower seeds, pumpkin seeds, hazelnuts, walnuts, etc.

Adding a tablespoon of soaked flax seeds or chia seeds to your smoothie, is another way to increase your fiber intake as well as give you a sensation of being full. Drink smoothies and green juices as needed and desired. The more you drink, the more you'll want. Your body will begin to ask for the greens!

The 'Get Your Feet Wet' Challenge

Simply follow the delicious recipes for making a daily smoothie to add to your current diet. Drink as much or as little as you like each day in addition to the other foods you would normally eat. If it feels right for you, consider becoming mindful of the feeling of physical hunger versus emotional hunger during your Challenge. One way to do this is to set specific times to eat during the day and make sure that you are good and hungry before you eat. This alleviates the constant need to decide whether or not to eat. Emotional eaters tend to want to eat at all times of the day, especially when stressed, anxious, lonely, bored, overwhelmed, sad, angry or feeling any other uncomfortable emotion. Food is comforting, so when we feel discomfort, we seek comfort. An emotional eater looks for comfort from food. As you can see, the desire to eat might have nothing to do with actual physical hunger. If this describes you, you are in good company because I too look to food for comfort when I feel uncomfortable. This is not a good or a bad thing. It is just a way many people cope. The key is to become aware of it. So, during this 'Get Your Feet Wet' Challenge, simply put your intention on becoming more aware of where your hunger is coming from. All cravings carry a message. They are in our lives to wake us up to what we feel we are missing. Consider tracking how you feel before, during and after you eat by keeping a journal. Often, emotional eaters feel frustrated and upset with themselves after eating, especially if they eat what they promised themselves not to eat, if they overeat or if they eat when they are not even hungry. Before eating, it can appear that the food will make you happy. After eating, the opposite is usually the outcome.

You might like to try my hypnosis exercise to end overeating to help you tune into your actual physical hunger and eat only when you are good and hungry and stop when you are just satisfied. You will find it at **www.mariarippo.com** under the 'Free Downloads' tab.

The Performance Enhancer

Taking a break from heavy exercise can be the most strengthening thing you can do as an athlete. Intense exercise is acid forming. It is a form of stress on the body. During The Challenge, your body is creating a more alkaline environment conducive to cleansing the body. For this reason, I find that intense exercise is best for times when you are not taking The Challenge.

If you do decide you'd like to continue with heavy exercise, simply make sure you are taking in enough calories to support your training. You can find healthy calories in the form of raw, soaked nuts and seeds, as well as avocados. Simply soak your nuts or seeds overnight and remove them from the water. You can rinse them and dehydrate in a dehydrator at 115° F or the lowest temperature in your oven with the door cracked open for 12 to 24 hours. Simply spread the nuts out on a baking sheet (if using oven) or tray in the dehydrator. Check after 12 hours and continue dehydrating until desired crispness is achieved.

For extra hydration, adding coconut water to your smoothies will greatly increase their hydration and mineral content. In addition, athletes may want to add a full meal or two to their day while on The Challenge. Choose a raw-food meal from this book or eat a meal you'd eat on a non-Challenge day, but leave out any processed food, sugar, table salt or pasteurized dairy.

Just remember that if you are going to exercise vigorously, it is imperative to get enough calories to support your body. Try to keep your meals to protein, healthy fat and vegetables.

Consider adding some protein powder to your smoothies. I like **Omega Nutrition's Pumpkin Seed Protein powder**. Coconut oil is another important addition, as this healthy fat will act as fuel for your body. **Bee pollen** is another healthy addition as it contains 22 amino acids, making it a complete protein. Local pollen is always best as it helps the most with allergies and immunity. If you have bee allergies, this is probably not the product for you. Check with your doctor. It also known for it's health and longevity benefits along with immune enhancing properties.

It would be wise to add some **bone broth** to your Challenge as well. Bone broth is rich in collagen, making it great for the joints. It is a rich source of protein and minerals, all-important for muscle recovery and building. It is very hydrating as well. See page 50 for my bone broth recipe or visit **www.mariarippo.com**.

Tips for Pregnant and Nursing Moms

Although you will need to check with your physician first, there are some things to consider if you'd like to join The Challenge while pregnant or nursing. In my opinion, this is not a time to do a full cleanse. During a body cleanse, you will be releasing a considerable amount of toxins, which can be released into your milk, if nursing. In both cases, getting enough calories to support your baby is also important. What you might consider is going off of all processed foods, table salt, white flour (and possibly all grains) and pasteurized dairy products excluding yogurt or kefir. Feel free to add as many smoothies as you feel good drinking as long as this is acceptable to your doctor or midwife. Also, include meals with a healthy balance of protein, fat, fruits and vegetables. Be extra careful about adding any herbs, supplements or other extras to your diet and always check with your physician before doing so. Many herbs are contraindicated during pregnancy or when nursing.

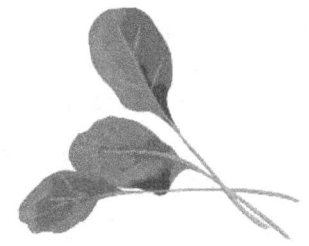

CHAPTER 5
One Day at a Time: Everything You Need to Conquer The Challenge

In this section, I will discuss different aspects of The Challenge that may or may not apply to you. Feel free to skip through any parts that you choose not include in your Challenge. I have also included a "Journaling" section. If you prefer to skip this section, please feel free! Just know that it may be very helpful in getting you through the entire Challenge.

> *Accept challenges, so that you may feel the exhilaration of victory. – George S. Patton*

Day 1

Upon waking, before you even sit up, I invite you to consider thinking of the three things in your life you are most thankful for. Be thankful that you are about to increase your energy level and health in dramatic ways. Be thankful that you *do* have the ability to stick with this. You *do*. You *can* do this and after trudging up hill for a little while, you'll be soaring like you may never have soared before. Step on the scale and measure your waist if tracking your progress in this manner is helpful. At the end of the challenge, you can re-measure and see your progress. You might want to take a picture, especially of your face because there will be a noticeable change!

Tea Time

Drink up to a liter of pure, room temperature or warm water with some fresh squeezed lemon juice and a teaspoon of sole each day. It is very important to drink a lot of water during this Challenge. Good hydration will help your body flush away the toxins that it releases as it burns extra fat. Listen to your body and drink water when you feel thirsty. Drink some ginger tea throughout the day as well. Add a little fresh lemon juice and stevia to it if you like. A cup of warm tea can do wonders as far as comforting a hungry tummy. You may add cinnamon as well. Cinnamon is a great addition because it helps with appetite control and is a blood sugar stabilizer. Have a cup of broth, if you prefer, or in addition to tea.

The Smoothie

Visit the recipe section in Chapter 6 and choose a smoothie recipe for today's "meals." You may also decide to make up your very own creation, and that is a great idea as well. Make 70 ounces of smoothie all at once for convenience. This also ensures that when you get hungry, your smoothie is ready for you. Try to drink about 16 ounces every three or four hours. Cut up some vegetables and fruit to take with you for the day. I prefer to munch on celery, cucumber, tomato, carrot, apples, pears, jicama, etc. Preparing your entire day's worth of food in the morning makes The Challenge simple and efficient. Remember that you are totally free to eat some soaked nuts or some guacamole or even an avocado with lemon juice, Celtic salt and some cayenne pepper. Just be careful, because if weight-loss is your goal, you will want to keep your calories to a minimum. The more you eat, the slower your body will cleanse too.

What to Expect Today

From the moment you were born and first drank milk from your mother's breast or from a warm bottle, you were comforted by food and nourishment. It is a fact of life: food *is* one of life's greatest pleasures. Food is comforting. Food brings people together. Food is part of how we identify ourselves. It is necessary for our survival and each one of us has a strong relationship to the food we eat. Not eating food may cause discomfort, fairly, severe discomfort in some, like me. Today, when it is mealtime and you smell the food that those around you are eating, it is normal to desire to eat with them. Know that as soon as you are finished with this healthy Challenge, you *will* be eating again. You are simply refraining from food for a short time and this will be over before you know it. You will be so glad for this bit of suffering when you have accomplished your goal, for suffering is the greatest catalyst for change.

If it helps, you can write down the foods you miss most today. You may notice that all of a sudden, every fast food joint you pass will beckon you to come and eat. You may turn on the TV and notice how many food commercials are there to tempt you. Your senses will be heightened and you may experience extreme temptation to eat. This temptation will become diminished with each day you conquer. By the tenth day, many people decide to stay on The Challenge longer than they had planned because they feel so good and no longer have a desire to eat those foods that keep them overweight, tired and unmotivated.

It can be helpful, when you have completed The Challenge, to see all the food you would have eaten and how it may have made you feel had you eaten it. By the ninth or tenth day, it is very common to feel a major difference in your energy levels. You may feel mad at yourself for having committed to this when it's dinnertime and you sit at the table with your smoothie. You may even be in quite a bad mood. These are *very* normal emotions to feel. Take some deep breaths and remember 'why' you are doing this and focus on how this will become part of your story of success in 10 short days. Let your family or friends know that this is temporary. Ask for their support. Try to get to bed early. Tomorrow is a new day and the scale, if you choose to weigh in, will be on your side!

If you feel depressed, I want you to know that I felt depressed for two months when I first went on a raw food diet. I realized how much I had been getting my comfort from food instead of dealing with my emotions. It is *very* normal for this to happen; so if and when it does, know that you are not alone. Food is comforting after all, and it is an easy way for us to numb our stresses, etc. We tend to use food to self-medicate. When we take away the comfort we get from food, we may be left with many emotions we have not yet dealt with. That may sound real strange and may not apply to you. I have food addiction and emotional eating-type tendencies so I experienced this in a strong way. Others may have a totally different experience. My husband felt angry at dinnertime the first time he did The Challenge. Be okay with it, if this happens to you. It's normal! Telling yourself that this is just a craving and that you are accustomed to eating for comfort, that the craving will pass and that you are going to find something else to do until it does, is very helpful. I even like to look at the clock and see how long it takes to pass, making it a game. The more you do this, the stronger you will become at not succumbing to cravings that do not serve you well.

Journaling

Gratitude is the antidote for depression. Practice the virtue of being thankful for what you **do** have.

Today, write down all the things you can think of that you are thankful for.

_____

_____

_____

_____

_____

_____

_____

_____

_____

_____

_____

_____

_____

_____

Day 2

As you did yesterday, upon waking, before you even sit up, think of the three things in your life you are most thankful for. Be thankful that you made it one day towards increasing your energy level and health in dramatic ways. Be thankful that you *do* have the ability to stick with this. You *do*. If you wish, step on the scale and see what happened yesterday. In 24 hours, you may have eliminated one, five or even more pounds of extra weight. Congratulations! Even if you do not see a difference on the scale, trust that your body *will* change. Know that you will likely feel tired today, especially as you near dinnertime. If you can, take a quick nap. If not, go to bed as early as possible. Your body may require extra sleep for a few days. It is hard at work burning fat, releasing and disposing of toxins and making repairs where necessary. Keep up the good work.

Tea Time

Like yesterday, have a cup of ginger tea or a glass of water with some fresh squeezed lemon juice upon rising. Add stevia if you like it sweet. Drink a few glasses of water to replace what was lost during the night. It is very important to drink plenty of water during this Challenge. This will help your body to flush away the toxins that it releases as it burns extra fat. Drink as much tea as you like today. It will really help keep your mind off of the food you have eliminated from your diet. Alternatively, start your day with a cup of warm broth.

The Smoothie

Choose your fruit and vegetables for today's smoothie. Mix up 70 ounces of smoothie like yesterday and remember to pack up some fresh fruit and veggies to snack on throughout the day.

What to Expect Today

If you have chosen to weigh yourself, after stepping on the scale, you may feel elated. You worked hard – you deserve it! Your hunger pangs may be more evident today. It's okay. They will subside in another day or two. Just munch on some veggies or an apple. Eat an avocado with some lemon juice, salt and cayenne pepper. If you are super hungry, mix up some more smoothie. Drink tea or broth throughout the day. After today, you'll be more than half way through the hardest part! Focus on your "why."

That which you resist, persists. If you give your energy to what you "cannot" eat, you will have given that energy away and will not have it for yourself. If you are thinking obsessively about what you are *not* eating and wish you *were*, try to find something else to occupy your mind. If you are simply bored, think about your passions in life. What gets you more excited than anything else? For me, it's studying about guiding myself and others through the process of transformation. For you, it may be creating a work of art, making a beautiful dress, fixing something, building something, volunteering, helping others, scrapbooking or fishing. Whatever it is that you can do that will occupy your mind in a positive way, something you look forward to doing and requires mental energy, will help to take your mind off of the hunger and temptations that you may experience. Figure out a way to start a new project in the area of your passion. If you do not have a passion, try finding something you can do for another person that would really make a difference in their life. This may bring you greater joy than anything you can do for yourself! You could set out to do something nice for someone else anonymously *everyday*!

> *Life is a paradise for those who love many things with a passion. – Leo Buscaglia*

Journaling

List making is the antidote for disorganization. Every day while on the fast, get up five minutes early and make a list of what you plan to accomplish for the day.

It is a good idea to have a master list of everything you would like to accomplish in life, including those things surrounding your passions. Look at it once a week or once a month. You can take things from this list to add to your weekly to-do list. It is good to keep track of what you would like to achieve in your life. Without making a conscious note of it, it likely will not get done. On the other hand, if you consciously plan to do something, you likely will! Make a to-do list for today and begin to work on your master list. It's a good idea to keep this in a notebook where you may refer to it and add to it as often as you like.

_____

_____

_____

_____

_____

_____

_____

_____

_____

_____

_____

_____

_____

_____

> *Take time to laugh, it is the music of the soul. – Unknown*

Day 3

Again, before getting out of bed, think of the three things in your life you are most thankful for. Be thankful you are in a place that allows you to take such a remarkable Challenge. Set your mind into a place of real gratitude. If you are struggling in your life, find three things you can be thankful for, even if it is the same three things every day. I know that when my husband and I were really struggling, I would practice truly being thankful that I had a roof over my head, water to drink and vegetables in my garden to feed my family. One way to find things to be thankful for is to think of what it might be like if you lost certain things. We were at a place at one time where it really was possible to not have a roof over our head, let alone a garden in the yard. This helped me to realize how truly blessed I was even if all my clothes were hand-me-downs from years prior and I didn't have an extra dime to spend. I became incredibly thankful that my children had heat, food and water! I was able to let go of the fact that they didn't have dance lessons, gymnastics, tai kwon do, etc. They had our love and the necessities, and I knew that those could not be taken away. It's amazing not to have to live on the street when you are in desperate circumstances. It has a way of drastically changing your perspective. So, another thing to be thankful for are the lessons that adversity teaches you.

Tea Time

By now, you may have a totally new relationship with tea or broth. Hopefully you are drinking tea all throughout the day and it has become a great comfort to your less-than-full tummy! Keep drinking your herbal and cleansing teas. A squeeze of lemon in each cup adds an extra punch of detoxification, vitamin C and refreshment.

The Smoothie

By now, you are getting acquainted with how the fruits and greens go together for the smoothie. Mix up your smoothie for the day and grab those munchies to take along. Consider meeting a friend, who is also doing The Challenge, for "lunch" today.

What to Expect Today

You are getting very close to a feeling of utter elation and clear mindedness. Remember today, in order to take your focus *off* of food, put your focus onto something that delights you, something you look forward to. Anticipate getting your energy back and your mind cleared up of the clutter that comes when we feel "out of control" with the cravings that can sometimes consume a good amount of mind share. Take a walk when others are eating. Know that you can and will persevere today! Remind yourself that taking time to cleanse and break away from all those tempting foods is just for a time. It will help you gain self-control again and allow you to experience the energy you feel when you do *not* eat those foods. This is a great motivator for you the next time you are confronted with a decision of whether or not to eat a certain food. Many times, I ask myself, "Is it more worth it to have a few moments of satisfaction as I consume this food, or is it more worth it to have the extra energy I will experience from making a different choice?" This is a decision only you can make for yourself, but it is a choice that often steers me to the celery instead of the bag of chips. I *love* to feel good!

Don't Quit

Author Unknown

When things go wrong, as they sometimes will,
When the road you're trudging seems all uphill,
When the funds are low, and the debts are high,
And you want to smile, but you frown a bit,
Rest if you must, but don't you quit.

Life is strange with its twists and turns,
As every one of us sometimes learns,
And many a failure turns about,
When he might have won had he stuck it out,
Don't give up though the pace seems slow,
You may succeed with another blow.

Success is failure turned inside out,
The silver tint of the clouds of doubt,
And you can never tell how close you are,
It may be near when it seems so far,
So stick to the fight when you're hardest hit,
It's when things seem worst
That you must not quit.

Finding Your Purpose

Find your definite purpose. According to Napoleon Hill, author of the classic **Think and Grow Rich**, this is the main action a person must take in order to be successful in attaining a goal. Begin with the end in mind.

Focus on what you plan to accomplish in this life. What is your purpose here? Try to narrow down where exactly it is that you are planning to go. This will take some time, so maybe just jot down some notes today and then come back to it later. For health and vitality, it is of utmost importance to know where you are headed, why you are here, what your purpose is. If you understand the importance of your unique existence on this planet, your body will function more optimally than if you feel despair and hopelessness, which tells your body it is time to stop living.

According to David Servan – Schreiber, MD, PhD and author of the international bestseller, **Anti-Cancer: A New Way of Life**, "When the … person gives up, feeling that life is no longer worth living, the immune system lays down its arms as well." Schreiber also notes that alternatively when one rediscovers the will to live often cancer turns toward healing. If your body understands how important it is to live, if your inner fire is stoked, your body systems will work hard to provide the energy necessary for health and vitality. If you feel hopeless, despairing and totally overwhelmed, that can give your body the message that it is time to stop living, which may bring you closer towards degeneration. Healing in this area often requires the guidance of a coach or therapist, which was true in my case.

The most common thing I find when working with clients is that people have not found their purpose and they don't know how to find it. I was forty before I began to know what my purpose was. Some people are seventy when they find it. If this describes you, you might like to say something like this to yourself right now: "Even though I don't know what my true purpose is, I love and accept myself anyway. Even though I feel foolish for not even knowing what my purpose is, I deeply and completely love and accept myself anyway. I completely accept myself and am open to finding my purpose." Take a few deep breaths and truly mean it. Compassion and acceptance for self are an integral part of moving forward.

When we are living in our purpose, we love what we are doing. Maybe we don't love every minute of it. We surely are growing and growing pains can be challenging, but we feel fulfilled and we have a knowing that we are using our most natural gifts to serve humanity.

---

[59] Servan-Schreiber, D. *Anticancer, a new way of life*. New York, NY: Penguin Group, 2008. Print.

Here are some important questions to ask yourself, if you'd like to know your purpose:

- If time and money were not an issue, what would I be doing?

- If I had a week off, what would I do with my time?

- What is something you do in your life that you can't imagine *not* doing?

- If you could sit for hours and talk about anything, what would it be?

- What do you do that you regularly receive compliments about?

- Is there something you love so much to do or to have that you are fine paying for the privilege of having/doing it?

- What do you daydream about doing?

- If I didn't have to do what I am going to do today, what would I do instead?

- If I could change one thing, one meaningful thing in my life, what would it be?

- What responsibilities/roles do I most enjoy and which do I least enjoy?

- If you had your dream job, what would it be?

- If all the experiences you've had in life were specifically designed to prepare you for your purpose, what would you say your life experiences have prepared you for?

- What are some of your most significant/memorable life experiences?

- What do you do that you are most recognized for?

- Who has been the greatest influence in your life?

- Have you taken a personality test? I use the Enneagram from a book called ***The Enneagram Made Easy*** or the Myers Briggs Type Indicator test. I find it incredibly enlightening to know your type and your unique gifts.

> *Whatever the circumstances of your life, the understanding of your type can make your perceptions clearer, your judgments sounder, and your life closer to your heart's desire.* – Isabel Briggs Myers

Another incredible tool I've found helpful is to have a natal chart reading. This is a very scientifically based way of looking at where and when you were born and where the planets were specifically at that time and place. This dictates much about who you are! I used to think it was non-sense until I had it done and I learned so much about myself that I concluded there must be a system to our personality types that is bigger than simple chance. I believe the Creator uses a very organized system for 'typing' us humans☺

The natal chart reader I use has been very instrumental in helping me see my gifts and more importantly, believe in my unique gifts. She has also helped me find the confidence to step out of my comfort zone to use them! You can use her services too. Her name is Liz Lyle, Astrological Counseling, **star.wise@earthlink.net**, 206-282-3212.

- What does your personality type make you good at?
- When your friends call on you, what do they ask of you? Are you one to hold a space for people, do they confide in you, do you bring the solution, create a distraction, bring food, listen, who are you to your friends?
- Do you have causes you support?
- Are you the one to get people together to support a cause?
- Are you the one people can count on to organize the details?
- What is your passion?
- If you had one year to live, what would you do?
- If this were your last day, what would you do?
- What do you do that you get lost in? When you do it, does time fly and you don't even know where it went?
- If you could change one thing in the world, what would it be?
- What excites you more than anything else?
- What makes you cry?

- What makes you laugh?

- What gives you joy?

- What do you ache for?

- What are willing to look like a fool for?

- What are you willing to disappoint another for in order to be true to yourself?

- What sustains you, makes you tick?

- When you come to the end of your life, is there something you would wish you had taken a risk for and might regret it if you didn't?

- If failure were not a possibility, what would you try?

- What do you love to learn about?

Look at your answers to the above questions. What purpose do your answers point to?

You express life in a way no other human being on the planet expresses it. Your job is to find the unique gifts, abilities and ways about you that are different than all other human beings. No other human grew up in your family, has had the trials you've had or the experiences you've had. You are unique and the wisdom *you* have is unique from every other individual on the planet. You might start by believing the truth in this.

> *The greater danger for most of us is not that our aim is too high and we miss it, but that it is too low and we reach it. – Michelangelo*

Journaling

Below, write your thoughts about your purpose on your journey here on planet Earth.

_____

_____

_____

_____

_____

_____

_____

_____

_____

_____

_____

_____

_____

_____

_____

Day 4

By now, you are probably used to the morning routine of lemon water and tea or broth. Are you beginning to feel more energy? You may or may not be. There is even a possibility that you may become sick with a cold or the flu. These are simply detoxification mechanisms for your body. If you do become sick or are extra tired, these are _great_ signs. They simply mean that your body has the message that it surely is time to rid itself of excess toxins. This is exciting because once the toxins are released, you are well on your way to experiencing a level of energy that you may never have felt before. This is a good time to remember that if you have not followed The Challenge exactly, relax! This is not a perfection contest. Just get right back on track and encourage yourself. Be kind to yourself. Your Self needs your support. Too often, we beat ourselves down, and it's a good lesson to learn to be kind to you! You are working hard. Pat yourself on the back. You are so close to feeling better than you have possibly ever felt before. Keep up the good work. Remember to find three things that you are thankful for and say them out loud. Are you beginning to truly feel more grateful for your life?

The Smoothie

Choose the smoothie you'll make today and pack up your munchies.

What to Expect Today

If you are excited about your results, be thankful. You have really made some headway. Great work! If you are really struggling, know that you are normal. You have made a "crazy" decision to clean out your system and stay away from so many of your favorite foods. That is a major change, and you *are* doing it! Keep going. Today will be the last of the *very* uphill days. You *can* do it and it will "magically" become easier from here on out. I'm sure the scale has become your friend by now if you have chosen to step on it, and it will continue to be a constant reminder of the positive changes this Challenge is bringing to you.

> *Courage and perseverance have a magical talisman, before which difficulties disappear and obstacles vanish into air. –*
> *John Quincy Adams*

Journaling

Be kind to yourself. Are there areas in your life where you are too hard on yourself? Do you need to be forgiven or to forgive yourself or others? Are you harboring bitterness that needs to be let go of? Where can you have more compassion for yourself?

Forgiveness is *not* about approving of another's behavior and forgetting what happened. Forgiveness is about releasing yourself from the prison that lack of forgiveness and resentment puts *you* in. Forgiveness is about releasing yourself from the bitterness you harbor towards another. Bitterness and resentment hold us captive and often do not cause suffering to another as we may think it will. Today, consider releasing yourself from the prison of resentment and bitterness. Forgiveness does not mean accepting hurtful behavior. It is about acknowledging it and how it affected you and then letting it go. Fred Luskin, Associate Professor of transpersonal psychology at Sofia University and Director of the Forgiveness Project at Standford University, offers some practical advice about forgiveness. He says that in order to forgive, we first must grieve the offense. It is imperative to first, acknowledge the harm done. Next, one must *feel* the pain, sadness, fear, shame, anger or trauma experienced from the offense. He says not to forget the event, but rather, transform our emotions attached to the event, to see if from a different perspective. The third step is to stop keeping the event a secret. Our connection to others is central to healing and being able to trust another to tell them our hurtful secrets is an important aspect of forgiveness. It helps us feel supported and not alone in our suffering. He also notes that telling everyone of our grievances, can be further damaging and to only share with a select few people that can be trusted. When one does not have someone to go to in confidence, it is advisable to go to a therapist or a 12-step program, the important aspect being letting go of the shame that is stored inside.

---

[60] Luskin, Fred. "What is Forgiveness?" *Greater Good: The Science of a Meaningful Life.* August 19, 2010. University of California, Berkeley. September 24, 2012.

A possible conversation with oneself regarding forgiveness might look something like this: "_____ happened. I am so sad (angry, ashamed, afraid, etc.) about it. Even though I am so sad (angry, ashamed, afraid, etc.) about _____, I completely and deeply love and accept myself anyway. I love and accept myself with all my imperfections. I'm so sad (angry, ashamed, afraid) that _____ happened. I haven't even shared it with anyone. I'm too ashamed/afraid. I have been so resentful because of _____ because I wanted to protect myself from having _____ happen again. It's not because I am despicable, I haven't forgiven because I didn't feel safe. Forgiveness feels scary to me. I feel _____ (scared, unworthy, like I don't matter, angry, ashamed, etc.). Why did _____ happen to me? It makes me so angry I want to scream. (Go ahead and scream if you feel like it or hit a pillow.) Of course I feel this way. Anyone would feel how I feel if _____ happened. It's so normal to feel _____. What if there is an important lesson for me to learn from this? What if I could let this resentment (bitterness, shame, anger, fear) go? How would my life be then? What if _____ was necessary for me to learn something I couldn't have learned any other way? What if I stopped blaming _____? What if I just focused on how it has made me feel and what it made me believe about myself? What if what I am believing about myself isn't true? What if there is another way for me to see it? What if I could say, "I forgive you" and "I will not allow this to happen to me again to the best of my ability. I don't deserve to be treated that way. I am valuable. I can protect myself even if I let go of this bitterness. I choose to forgive myself. I choose to forgive _____. I choose to take the lessons I've learned and accept different treatment from others. I bless _____ as they learn the lessons they need to learn, even though I do NOT excuse their behavior. It feels good to let go. I feel calm. I breathe deeply. I am at peace. I deeply and completely love and accept myself and allow myself to learn as all humans must do." Now take a deep breath and see if you feel differently about what happened. If you'd like to take it a step further, recreate the scenario in your mind. Go ahead get creative. Create a new outcome. Your mind doesn't know the difference between what is real and what is imaginary. Often, the grief period takes longer than the two minutes you just spent. Allow it to take as long as it needs and seek the guidance of a professional if necessary. Above all, honor your emotions instead of fighting them or pretending they do not exist.

> *To err is human, to forgive, Divine. –*
> *Alexander Pope*

Write a little bit about your relationships with yourself and those near to you. What areas are you struggling with? What areas are you thankful for? Write down some areas that may need attention.

_____

_____

_____

_____

_____

_____

_____

_____

_____

_____

_____

_____

_____

_____

Day 5

Congratulations! You have made it through the most challenging few days! You are becoming stronger, more energetic and you may have lost a decent amount of weight by now. I'm thrilled for you. Make yourself an extra delicious smoothie today to celebrate. Drink your smoothie in a martini glass or other celebratory vessel. Have a bowl of my healthy ice cream too. You deserve it. If dinnertime is especially difficult for you, always drink a smoothie while others eat, have some tea or go for a walk.

Tea Time

Have your cup of tea/broth and drink it too! Make sure you add fresh lemon juice for extra cleansing. As you drink your beverage, remind yourself of your "why." Why are you really doing this? Envision making it to day ten. How are you going to feel? What will you do with all that extra energy? How will your clothes fit differently? What kind of changes will you have made in your quality of life? Take a minute to contemplate these things.

The Smoothie

Make your daily smoothie and pack your snacks. Consider switching the snacks you bring along each day.

What to Expect Today

Now that you have made it this far, your possible anxiety about not eating should be subsiding. This is a good time to start on that organizing project and setting goals for the year. Now that your mind is beginning to clear up, you will be able to think more clearly about your goals. Go ahead and write down your short-term goals, such as plans for eating a more healthy diet and being consistent with your exercising. I haven't mentioned that one of the side-effects of cleansing your body is that you may mysteriously begin to cleanse your life. Before you know it that desk will be in order, the laundry will all be done and your house will be neat and tidy. I keep a "fasting" journal because when my mind clears up I begin to think clearly about the things in my life that are important to me. I begin to realize things I had not seen before. It seems every year I see a new major area that needs some overhauling. When I fast I don't need as much sleep, so I end up writing out ways to improve these areas.

For example, I spent one year learning how to be organized. I read books and talked to people who are more efficient than me. I spent a year figuring out ways to be more efficient and it has really made a difference, and yes, I still get disorganized and just keep practicing getting reorganized. Next, I became aware of the hurtful and negative way that I was speaking to myself. I read books on this subject regarding how to actively change my self-talk. This has dramatically affected so many areas of my life. I realized the bitterness and lack of forgiveness I was harboring. My family has especially benefitted. Now when they come home, they are greeted by a mother who feels truly blessed that she has her family. In the past, I spent all day complaining silently about my life. I learned to turn my thoughts around and think in new way. I continue to practice gratitude in these areas and of course, I am still human and not perfect at it.

> *Finally, brothers, whatever is true, whatever is noble, whatever is right, whatever is pure, whatever is lovely, whatever is admirable—if anything is excellent or praiseworthy—think about such things. – Philippians 4:8, NIV*

> *You have not lived today until you have done something for someone who can never repay you. – John Bunyon*

Consider being open to hearing and seeing the areas of your life that you might need to work on. I invite you to consider being OK that you have areas that need work because if you did not, you'd be the only one. We *all* have them. Oftentimes we are afraid to take a good look at these areas and would like to think we've got it all figured out. But none of us do. The only way to begin healing and moving forward is to know that every person on the planet has areas of their lives that they would rather no one know about. It is very freeing to begin to see these areas in ourselves and to even talk to others about them. The most important thing is to have compassion for ourselves as we learn.

> *In reading the lives of great men, I found that the first victory they won was over themselves…self-discipline with all of them came first. – Harry S. Truman*

Journaling

Listen to your self-talk today. What kinds of things are you telling yourself throughout the day? What kinds of things is your Self telling you?

Write down the conversations you are having with yourself today. Is your voice inside mainly positive or negative? Do you have an attitude of gratitude or of criticism, helplessness and fear?

> *The strangest secret in the world is that you become what you think about. – Earl Nightengale*

_____

_____

_____

_____

_____

_____

_____

_____

_____

_____

_____

_____

_____

_____

Day 6

Only four more days. You're so close. You are going to make it to the end! Imagine how you will look and feel. Are you experiencing greater efficiency of your mind? This is my favorite part of fasting and cleansing. By about day six, my mind becomes so clear, I can think and prioritize in a way that I do not experience otherwise.

Tea Time

Drink your morning tea and continue to drink as much as you like throughout the day. You may find yourself needing less and less tea each day. Listen to your body, and drink the amount that seems to work for you.

The Smoothie

Mix, blend, pack and go!

What to Expect Today

You may now have passed the stage where you experienced anxiety as a result of your lack of food intake. It's a good idea to take a look at your experience to find out if you use food for reasons other than nourishment. To an extent, we all do this, some more than others. Food is very comforting and oftentimes a person will eat, instead of recognizing and dealing with feelings of fear, anxiety, stress, helplessness, anger, sadness, etc. This is called "self-medicating." I know I do it. I've learned to ask myself: "Am I physically hungry or is this soul hunger?" When you feel the urge to eat, try to recall how long it has been since your last meal. If it has been less than three hours, you may have a desire to eat in order to fill a void that you are not even aware of. When this happens to me, I stop and think about what is really going on. Am I stressed out, angry, sad, bored? If I can discover which emotion I'm feeling, then I can begin to validate that the emotion is stressful, angering or sad, etc. It is OK to feel these feelings. Emotions, in and of themselves, are not good or bad. They are simply neutral, and it is OK to feel them. It is important to be aware of them because once we are aware of them, we can begin to figure out how to change the situation or deal with it in a healthy manner. If we try to pretend they are not there, we'll never be able to do anything about them and they will eat at us, literally. Emotions are powerful messengers and they will persist until we hear the message.

> *If you wish success in life, make perseverance your bosom friend, experience your wise counselor, caution your elder brother and hope your guardian genius. – Joseph Addison*

Journaling

> *If you fail to plan, then plan to fail. – Unknown.*

Take some time to write out the positive lifestyle changes you plan to make once your Challenge is complete.

What is your plan for eating and exercise when you have successfully completed this Challenge? You may decide to drink a green smoothie or green juice every day. You may want to add a big salad to your lunch menu. It is best to decide what you are going to do instead of what you are not going to do. Decide on the things you plan to add into your lifestyle that will be healthy habits. Now is the best time to implement these changes, as your body will crave good foods. In Chapter 8, I offer some recipes to try. If you prefer to eat a meat-based diet, check out **www.marksdailyapple.com** by Mark Sisson. One of my all-time favorite books on health is ***The Body Ecology Diet***. I also recommend Paul Chek's ***How to Eat, Move and Be Healthy***. For a vegetarian plan, the Vegetarian Health Institute offers a free guide to vegetarian eating called ***The Secret to Being Fit Forever.*** You can find it free online at **www.veghealth.com/fit-forever/**.

_____

_____

_____

_____

_____

_____

_____

_____

_____

_____

_____

_____

_____

_____

Day 7

Hopefully you are experiencing some very positive results by now. How is your attitude?

> *A cheerful heart hath a continual feast. –*
> *Proverbs 15:15*

Tea Time

You may like to go out and get some interesting new flavors of tea to spice up your day a little. Just make sure the tea does not contain caffeine or added sugar. Organic herbs are preferable.

The Smoothie

Consider trying an interesting new combination of fruits in your smoothie today. Remember to pack up fresh fruit and veggies to nibble on.

What to Expect

Do you have experience with deep breathing? Deep breathing oxygenates your cells, which is important for all aspects of health. Deep diaphragmatic breathing calms the **nervous system** because the slow, rhythmic, deep breathing sends a message to the nerve endings on the floor of the brain that everything is all right and it's okay to relax. In a study conducted at Stanford University School of Medicine, shallow breathing was found to actually create **anxiety**. In the same way, slow, deep, rhythmic breathing can create relaxation. "An intimate connection exists between the mind and the breath." When we are disturbed emotionally, our breath is immediately affected such as when we hear a loud sound and are startled. Likewise, the breath influences the mind.

Deep, diaphragmatic breathing is very detoxifying because it oxygenates the blood, enabling the blood to detoxify the body more efficiently.

In order to practice deep breathing, find a comfortable, quiet, peaceful place to lie down or sit with your legs crisscrossed like a pretzel and back erect. This position works best if your knees are below your hips, so you may want to elevate your bottom to get comfortable. Your bed is a good spot if your room is tidy. Open a window to let in some fresh air. Close your eyes and rest for a minute. Now, breathe in through your nose to a count of eight. Count slowly. Place one hand on your chest and the other on your abdomen. Allow the air to bypass your chest and fill your abdomen like a balloon. Hold the breath for a count of eight if it is comfortable. Now exhale out of your mouth to a count of eight. Continue to breathe slowly in this manner. Think of a warm, sunny beach or other location that would be very relaxing. You can continue this breathing for five minutes or up to a half hour. Notice how it calms your entire being. You might just take a nap.

Journaling

Stop and reflect today. What are the reasons you decided to take The Challenge? What are some of the biggest obstacles you have overcome? Are you thrilled that you've made it a week on pure, healthy green smoothies? Congratulate yourself! This is quite an accomplishment!

---

[61] Appl Psychophysiol Biofeedback. 2007 Jun; 32(2):89-98. Epub 2007 May 23.

[62] Walters, Donald J. *The Art and Science of Raja Yoga*. Revised Edition. Nevada City, California: Crystal Clear Publishers, 2010. 61. Print.

Today, really take note of the positive changes you have experienced. Write down how differently you feel today, compared to one week ago.

_____
_____
_____
_____
_____
_____
_____
_____
_____
_____
_____
_____
_____
_____

> *Far better to dare mighty things, to win glorious triumph, even though checkered by failure, than to take rank with those poor spirits who neither enjoy much nor suffer much, because they live in the gray twilight that knows not victory, nor defeat.*
> — *Theodore Roosevelt*

Day 8

You're so close to the finish line. You can see it in the distance. What a way to kick start your week, your month, your year, your life! I hope you have worked through the journal and have given thought to some of these important considerations. Look back over your entries for this week. You may be making a daily to-do list. Continue this routine and watch it change your level of efficiency.

Tea Time

By now, you have grown accustomed to your morning tea/broth ritual. Enjoy a nice, warm refreshing cup this morning and throughout the day.

The Smoothie

Try making one of the Boutenko's smoothies today if you have not already. Remember to pack your snacks.

What to Expect

You will notice that you are not requiring quite as much smoothie on a daily basis. Keep drinking the same amount in order to keep your metabolism fired up. You may be experiencing a stronger desire to exercise, so make sure to fit it into your day. As your energy level increases, your body craves movement. Workouts help to cleanse and strengthen your system.

Journaling

If you are up for it, consider adding five minutes to your early morning routine. After you make your list for the day, take five minutes to reflect on your intentions for the day.

I like to pray. It helps me get my perspective in the right place. It calms me in areas of stress. Here's an example of a prayer that gets me in the right place as soon as I wake up:

> "Lord, today, give me the grace to trust in the plan You have for me. Allow me to know that I am exactly in the place You have put me right now. When my plans are thwarted or my day interrupted, let these be reminders to me that Your plan is the one I want to follow. When I feel weary, lift me up; when weak, give me strength; when I fear, impart trust to me. I give You this day to continue to write the story of my life. Allow me to see You in all things. Enable me to know my strengths and areas of challenge and to be content with the person You have made me. Help me to see where I can love more, give more, trust more, forgive more, to believe more. Help me to meet all those who cross my path just where they are, without judgment, but with kindness, understanding, love and compassion as I would have others do for me. "

And in the words of St. Francis:

> "…make me an instrument of peace. Where there is hatred, let me sow love. Where there is doubt, faith, where there is despair, hope. Where there is darkness, light. Where there is sadness, joy. Amen."

If this is something that would be helpful to you, write out a prayer or something that will remind you daily of the things you would like to be focusing on in your life.

I like to refer to this as "setting my perspective" for the day. It really helps me to remember the big picture in life and not to get so bent out of shape over all of the small obstacles that each day is sure to bring.

> *I hold a doctrine, to which I owe not much, indeed, but all the little I ever had, namely, that with ordinary talent and extraordinary perseverance, all things are attainable. –*
> *Sir T. F. Buxton*

_____

_____

_____

_____

_____

_____

_____

_____

_____

_____

_____

_____

_____

_____

_____

Day 9

Just imagine, tomorrow, one day from now, you will be able to say: "I did it!" By now it may even seem like you could keep going beyond the ten days you had planned to do. I hope you are full of energy and excitement. You may feel very excited about the thought that you will eat regular food again after tomorrow. An interesting phenomenon is that often a person gets to the point where they can eat, but they end up desiring to continue on The Challenge. Listen to your body. It will be speaking to you from a nourished standpoint. It will tell you what it wants to do. If you prefer to continue on your current path, check with your health care provider to make sure it's right for you.

Tea Time

Meet a friend for tea today. Tell someone what you've done. Live it up!

The Smoothie

Time your smoothie making today. See how long it takes you to make your entire day's worth of 'food.' The convenience of it may convince you to add these nutrition-packed drinks to your day every day from here on out! Mix up that smoothie and pack your munchies.

What to Expect

You may experience joy and contentment in a job well done today. You are nearing the attainment of quite a lofty goal. In what ways are you experiencing change? Often when we take on a difficult challenge, it has a way of transforming us in ways we never would have imagined. It is my hope that you have this experience.

How Well Do You Know Yourself?

It is a good idea, if you have not spent time getting to know you, to do so now. One reason it's important to take some time to really understand who you are is that you will be able to find out what your strengths and weaknesses are. The Myers-Briggs Type Indicator is a good place to start. Another helpful resource is a book called *The Enneagram Made Easy*. If we understand our strengths, we will be better equipped to move in a direction that utilizes them. When we understand our weaknesses we can create a tool bag to help us respond in healthy ways to the challenges and obstacles that are inevitable in life.

Journaling

Take time today to write down your strengths, as well as areas that are challenging. Usually, when we find things we are very strong in, we can see the exact opposite area that is a challenging part of who we are. So, every weakness is usually paired with an area of strength. Take some time to learn more about your personal strengths and weaknesses.

_____

_____

_____

_____

_____

_____

_____

_____

_____

_____

_____

_____

_____

_____

Day 10

Listen for the cosmic drum roll today! Congratulations! You've made it. You've done it. Imagine being introduced on stage today as the new _(your name here)_ . You truly have begun the process of becoming new as far as renewing your cells and being a totally rejuvenated person. Please write to me and tell me your story. I would love to hear about your experience. **maria@thegreensmoothiechallenge.com**

Tea Time

Toast to yourself this morning. What a milestone for you. What an amazing thing you have done for yourself! Great job! You did it.

The Smoothie

Re-create your own favorite smoothie from the last ten days or follow the recipe for the last day in my recipe section. Make sure to pour it into a celebratory glass and toast to your success. Cheers!

What to Expect

Utter elation! Amazement in your accomplishment! Superhuman powers! You may desire to continue your Challenge. This is a decision only you can make. Choose wisely! You may desire to completely change how you eat from now on. Many raw food chefs have lovingly offered recipes included in the recipe section of this book. I have provided information about each contributor so you may find more recipes. Experiment and have fun. Remember the difference living on live food for ten days has made for you. It is possible to feel this good on a regular basis by adding a large variety of living foods to your diet! Although I do not recommend a raw-food, vegan diet for the long term, these are some delicious and healthy recipes to include in a healthy, balanced diet. I have included suggestions for coming off The Challenge in Chapter 8. Begin now to plan what you will consume in the next few days as you slowly add food back into your regimen.

Journaling

Take time to reflect on your experience. Was it worthwhile for you? What did you get out of it? What were your favorite parts? What was the most challenging for you? Would you do this again? How do you feel and look differently?

Find your constitutional make-up. When we are working towards total health and wellness it is important to learn about our unique individual make-up. This will help us to better understand our personal nutritional needs. Ayurvedic medicine has an effective system for this which you can research online. You can find out what your **dosha** is and how to balance it at **doshaquiz.chopra.com**. There is also a helpful metabolic typing test you can take in a book called, ***How to Eat, Move and Be Healthy*** by Paul Chek of the Chek Institute. Understanding your constitutional type will assist you in knowing how to balance your intake of protein, fat, and carbohydrates as well as helping you to understand what times of day are best for your biggest meal. There is no diet that works for every person. We are all unique, and spending a little time figuring this out is very helpful. I offer metabolic type testing. Feel free to **book an appointment with me at http://www.mariarippo.com/book-an-appointment.html.**

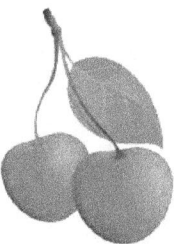

CHAPTER 6
The Green Smoothie Challenge Recipes

I dedicate this section to the Boutenko family. For without them, embarking on this life-altering adventure would be a distant thought still awaiting us.

Here are the same recipes I used to make the smoothies that enabled my husband to lose fifteen pounds in nine days! I included a tenth recipe for your tenth day as well. Simply follow one recipe per day, which will yield a day's worth of smoothies for one adult.

Helpful hints: When called for, I use Sweetleaf™ brand pure stevia extract. I also have tried the Pure Organic Stevia Leaf Extract from Trader Joe's, which includes a tiny scooper. KAL brand is good and also has a scooper. It is preferable to use a high-power blender like a Blendtec™.

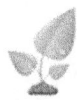

Peachy Keen

1 apple, quartered

½ cup (5 oz) grapes, frozen or fresh

1 cup (5 oz) frozen peaches

1 cup (5 oz) frozen strawberries

3 cups water

1½ leaves (4 oz) kale, de-stemmed

2 big handfuls (4 oz) spinach

4 cups water

2 tbsp flax or chia seeds

5 scoops stevia

Place fruit in blender with 3 cups of water and blend. Pour mixture into a large container. Place veggies into blender with 4 cups of water and blend. Add this to the fruit mixture. Add stevia and flax or chia seeds and mix it all up. Enjoy! Makes about 70 ounces total.

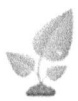

An Apple a Day

1 frozen banana (peeled before freezing)

1 apple, quartered

1½ cups frozen strawberries

3 cups water

2½ large curly leaves (6 oz) kale, destemmed

5 scoops stevia

2 packed cups (2.6 oz) baby salad greens

4 cups water

2 tbsp flax or chia seeds

Place fruit in blender with 3 cups water and blend. Pour mixture into a large container. Place veggies into blender with 4 cups water and blend. Add this to the fruit mixture. Add stevia flax or chia seeds and mix it all up. Enjoy! Makes about 70 ounces total.

Banana Berry Blast

1 apple, quartered

1 banana

1½ cups frozen mixed berries

2 cups water

2 large swiss chard leaves

2 handfuls spinach leaves

3 scoops stevia

2 tbsp flax or chia seeds

2 cups water

Place fruit in blender with 2 cups of water and blend. Pour mixture into a large container. Place veggies into blender with 2 cups of water and blend. Add this to the fruit mixture and mix it all up. Add stevia and flax or chia seeds. Enjoy! Makes about 70 ounces total.

You're a Peach

1 head romaine lettuce

1 handful spinach leaves

1 handful frozen peaches

1½ cups frozen mixed berries

2 ½ cups water

7 scoops stevia

1 tsp vanilla

5 shakes Celtic salt

2 tbsp flax or chia seeds

2 ½ cups water

Place fruit in blender with 2 ½ cups of water and blend. Pour mixture into a large container. Place veggies into blender with 2 cups of water and blend. Add this to the fruit mixture and mix it all up. Add salt and flax or chia seeds. Enjoy! Makes about 70 ounces total.

The Slurpy Smoothie

One day, I made a smoothie for Tobin, and my kids begged to try it—music to my ears. They loved it and said it tasted like a slurpy. Thus, the name.

8 leaves romaine lettuce

2 cups water

1 cup frozen peaches

1½ cups frozen mixed berries

2 tbsp flax or chia seeds

stevia to sweeten *(a little goes a long way!)*

2 cups water

Place fruit in blender with 2 cups of water and blend. Pour mixture into a large container. Place lettuce into blender with 2 cups of water and blend. Add this to the fruit mixture and mix it all up. Add stevia and seeds Enjoy! Makes about 70 ounces total.

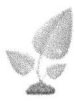

Tropical Sunshine

1 handful frozen pineapple chunks

1 frozen banana

1½ cups frozen mango chunks

1 cup frozen mixed berries

3 cups water

2 handfuls spinach leaves

3 handfuls baby spring mix salad greens

4 cups water

2 tbsp flax or chia seeds

Place fruit in blender with 3 cups of water and blend. Pour mixture into a large container. Place veggies into blender with 4 cups of water and blend. Add this to the fruit mixture and mix it all up. Add flax or chia seeds. Enjoy! Makes about 70 ounces total.

Almond Milk Elixir

20 oz almond milk*

4 cups water

Seeds from ½ of a pomegranate

1½ cups (6 oz) frozen mangoes

1 banana

1 cup (4.2 oz) frozen mixed berries

3 cups water

2 large (4.2 oz) leaves curly kale

2 heads of romaine hearts

2 tbsp flax or chia seeds

4 - 5 cups water

*To make almond milk, soak 1 cup of raw almonds in pure water over night. Rinse and strain water off. Place the almonds in a blender with 4 cups water. Blend for about 2 minutes. Pour milk through a **produce bag** (the produce department at your grocery store may carry these) or fine mesh strainer to remove the "pulp." Alternatively, use store-bought organic almond milk. (Almond milk recipe is also on page 124).

For the Smoothie: Remove seeds from the pomegranate. Add other fruits and fill blender with water (about 3 cups). Blend. Pour into container. Add greens to blender and fill with water (about 4 or 5 cups). Blend and add to fruit mixture. Enjoy!

My Daily Fare

1 apple

1 frozen banana

1½ cups mixed frozen berries

2 cups water

4 leaves kale

2 handfuls spinach

2 tbsp flax or chia seeds

2 cups water

Place fruit in blender with 2 cups of water and blend. Pour mixture into a large container. Place veggies into blender with 2 cups of water and blend. Add flax or chia seeds. Add this to the fruit mixture and mix it all up. Enjoy! Makes about 70 ounces total.

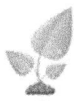

Berries, Mangoes and Pears, Oh My

1 pear

6 oz mangoes

1½ cups frozen strawberries

2 cups water

1 head romaine lettuce

2 tbsp flax or chia seeds

2 cups water

Place fruit in blender with 2 cups of water and blend. Pour mixture into a large container. Place veggies into blender with 2 cups of water and blend. Add this to the fruit mixture and mix it all up. Enjoy! Makes about 70 ounces total.

Celebration Smoothie!

¼ pomegranate

6 oz mangoes

5 oz pineapple

2 cups water

2 leaves kale

2 handfuls salad greens

2 cups water

Place fruit in blender with 2 cups of water and blend. Pour mixture into a large container. Place veggies into blender with 2 cups of water and blend. Add this to the fruit mixture and mix it all up. Enjoy! Makes about 70 ounces total.

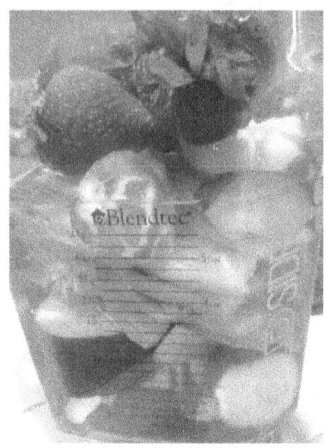

Maria's Daily Sunshine Smoothie

3 stalks celery

1 medium zucchini

½ large cucumber

1" piece of ginger

½ lemon or lime partially peeled

2" portion of aloe gel from a stalk of aloe

4 cups water

1 small peach

3 large strawberries

1 tbsp virgin coconut oil

2 scoops Omega Nutrition pumpkin seed protein powder

2 tsp bee pollen

Now if that is not an ahhhhh-mazingly healthy green smoothie recipe, I don't know what is!! This is also a perfect green smoothie challenge recipe!! If you like to add ground chia or flax seed, that is a perfect addition, as it will make the smoothie more filling and fiberous.

Maria's Thyroid Friendly, Sugar Free Green Smoothie

1 small zucchini

1 medium cucumber

3 stalks celery

1 small handful parsley

1 small handful cilantro

½ lemon, mostly peeled

1" piece of ginger

3 - 4 cups water

1 green apple, optional

1 tbsp coconut oil, optional

Fresh aloe, optional

Add berries or other fruit if that works for your body. I do not add fruit to mine. A little stevia should be okay if you need a sweetener.

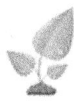

Green Juice Recipes

It would be very beneficial to include one green juice into your Challenge each day. These do require special equipment such as a juice extractor. I recommend using the **Breville®**, **Champion®** or **Hurom® juicers**. You may also make these in your blender and then simply strain them through a **nylon produce bag**.

Here are my favorite green juice recipes.

Simple Green Juice Recipe

1 cucumber

6 leaves of kale or romaine lettuce

3 stalks celery

Place ingredients through juicer and enjoy.

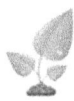

Fresh "V8" Juice

2 tomatoes, quartered

2 cloves garlic

½ green pepper

1 carrot

2 stalks celery

¼ bunch of spinach

¼ bunch of parsley

1 lemon

Cayenne pepper

Himalayan or Celtic salt

Run all ingredients through your juicer. Add cayenne pepper and Himalayan or Celtic salt to taste, if desired! Enjoy daily.

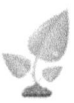

Green Juice with Ginger

6 leaves kale

1 cucumber

6 leaves romaine lettuce

1 lemon

1 finger of ginger root

3 stalks celery

Place ingredients through juicer and enjoy.

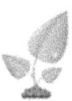

Green Juice with Sprouts

1 cucumber

3 stalks celery

6 leaves kale

1 bunch greens

1 handful sprouts of choice

1 handful parsley

Place ingredients through juicer and enjoy.

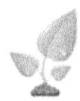

I am Healthy All-Green Energy Drink

This recipe is kindly contributed by Café Gratitude. With its inspiring environment and flavorful organic foods, the café was founded by Terces Engelhart with locations in San Fransisco, Berkeley, Marin and Los Angeles. The following recipe can be found in Terces' recipe book, *I Am Thankful*. In her book she tells of her own recovery from eating disorders, explains the amazing health benefits of raw foods and shares the café's trademark recipes. I highly recommend this book. It can be found in the online store of Café Gratitude.

8 oz cucumber juice

5 oz celery juice

3 oz kale juice

Splash of lemon juice

Pour fresh juices into a goblet, adding a splash of lemon at the end; garnish with a lemon wedge. We add 1 tablespoon of sole for extra flavor. Makes 16 ounces.

These are additional optional recipes for you to use freely while on The Challenge. These have been generously contributed for your enjoyment by the Boutenko family, Kevin and Annmarie Gianni and Clent Manich.

For the recipes that do not offer an amount of water to add, simply fill the blender with the ingredients and then add water to about half way up to the top of the ingredients; so half as much water as ingredients. That usually works perfectly!

Dancing Dandelion Smoothie by Igor Boutenko

3 cups freshly picked dandelion greens

2 cups apple juice

1 cup water

1 fresh mango

1 ripe peach

Place ingredients in blender and blend until smooth. Yields two quarts.

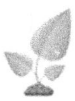

Morning Zing Smoothie by Sergei Boutenko

½ bunch of dandelion greens

2 stalks celery

½ inch piece of fresh ginger root

2 peaches

½ cup pineapple

Add ingredient to blender with desired amount of water. Blend and enjoy! Yields two quarts.

Wicked Watermelon Smoothie by Sergei Boutenko

4 cups fresh watermelon chunks, rind removed

1 banana

5 leaves romaine lettuce

juice of ½ lemon

Place ingredients in blender with desired amount of water and blend until smooth. Yields two quarts.

Memory Booster Brain Smoothie by *Valya Boutenko*

2 cups freshly picked purslane

1 organic cucumber with peel

1 lime, juiced

2 ripe pears

½ apple

2 cups water

Place ingredients in blender and blend until smooth. Yields two quarts.

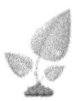

Maria's "Kid Approved" Green Smoothie!

½ cup frozen organic pineapple

6 or 7 strawberries

1 cup of fresh spinach

water to fill blender

1 tsp vanilla

Himalayan or Celtic salt to taste

Blend well in blender and serve immediately.

Kevin and Annmarie Gianni are the hosts of the daily Internet show *The Renegade Health Show*. Kevin is a health advocate, author, interviewer and film consultant. Annmarie has been involved in athletics and healthy living since childhood. She received her Sports Medicine degree from East Carolina University and now has an amazing skin care company, well worth checking out! To get their books and learn more about them or to download a free copy of Kevin's book, *High Raw*, visit **www.therenegadehealthshow.com**.

Kevin and Annmarie Gianni's Gingerly Sweet Smoothie

1 mango

1 handful of greens of your choice

1 lemon, with skin removed, keeping a little of the white

¼ inch piece of ginger, remove the skin

1 date

1 cup of coconut water

Blend and enjoy!

Clent Manich's Daily Favorite Smoothie

Because of the high content of greens in this recipe, Clent was able to lose a lot of weight. This recipe was kindly shared by **www.greensmoothierevolution.com**

1 big handful of mixed greens or organic baby salad greens

1 big handful of spinach

4 leaves of kale (and/or)

4 leaves of collard greens (and/or)

¼ bunch of dandelion greens

¼ bunch of parsley (and/or)

Handful of beet leaves (and/or)

1 banana

1 large tomato or 2 medium tomatoes

½ avocado

½ lemon squeezed

½ lime squeezed

1 apple

4 large strawberries

2 tbsp ground flaxseed

2 cups pure water

1 cup of ice

Blend it all in batches and pour it into one large container and shake well before drinking.

Robin's Creamsicle

Robin inspired many as she embarked on and completed a 40 day Green Smoothie Challenge while others were simply making it through only ten days. It made ten days seem like a short amount of time. Here she shares her favorite combo.

1 bunch on spinach

2 frozen bananas

1 orange

½ lime, juice only

½ lemon, juice only

½ inch piece Madagascar vanilla bean, seeds scraped into blender

1 tbsp raw agave nectar (I would prefer to use stevia as agave is very high in fructose)

1 cup of ice

Water if needed.

Combine ingredients, blend and enjoy.

Heather's Low Glycemic Spicy Smoothie

Heather became a big fan of The Challenge after many failed attempts at releasing weight and feeling healthy. She had even been to the doctor to see if he had any solutions for her lack of weight loss. After taking The Challenge and consistently releasing a half-pound per day for ten days, she was a believer and fast became one of my biggest fans. Here is her famous spicy smoothie.

Fill blender ⅔ full with spinach

½ avocado

½ a bunch of cilantro

1 medium jalapeno

1 granny smith apple

2-3 leaves kale or chard

Juice from ½ a lemon

pinch of salt

About 4 -5 cups of water depending on desired thickness.

Place all ingredients in blender and mix until smooth and delicious.

Non-Smoothie Recipes to Enjoy
While Taking The Challenge

Almond Milk

Almond milk itself is a delectable treat. Simply place two scoops of stevia into a glass and fill the glass with this tasty drink.

<u>The night before you plan to make the milk:</u>

Place 1 cup of raw, organic almonds into a bowl.

Cover the almonds with pure water and allow to sit over night.

<u>To make your milk:</u>

Simply rinse and drain the almonds.

Place them in your blender and fill the blender with water. Blend well.

Strain the almond milk through a sprouting bag, cheesecloth or a strainer to remove the pulp. *(Save the pulp to use in Maria's Festive Seed Cheez recipe on page 146).*

This will give you beautiful white milk that you can drink or use in many of my recipes, including ice cream.

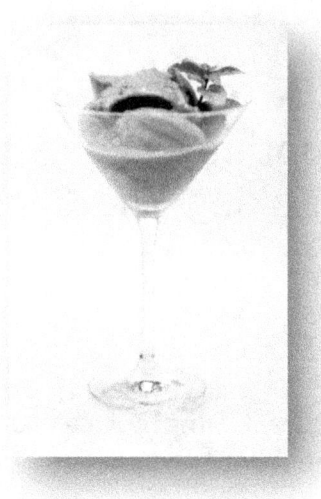

Strawberry Delight Ice Cream

12 ounces almond milk (recipe on page 124)

1 ½ handfuls frozen strawberries

¼ cup Pure birch xylitol

1 tsp vanilla

8 scoops stevia

Celtic salt, to taste

About 14 ice cubes

Place all ingredients in blender and blend.

Continue adding ice cubes until it has the ice cream consistency you are looking for. If you have a **Blendtec™ blender**, you can simply blend on the ice cream setting.

Maria's Enzyme Rich Avocado Soup

2 cups avocado

2 cups water

½ cup fresh cilantro

½ cup fresh parsley

1 cup celery

2 roma tomatoes

½ cup sundried tomatoes (soaked in water for 8 hours) use the dried kind, not soaked in olive oil

¼ onion

¼ tsp cayenne pepper

½ cup spinach

¼ cup fresh lemon juice

If you don't have the sundried tomatoes, just make the soup without them. Place all ingredients in blender and blend until smooth and creamy. You may chop up some of the veggies instead of blending them if you prefer your soup to be chunky. Blend for an extra-long time to warm or place on stovetop and blend until just warm to the touch, less than 118° F to keep all enzymes and nutrients in tact.

Maria's Heavenly Chocolate Shake

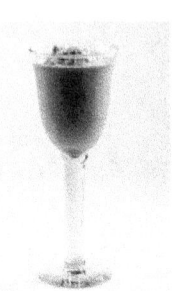

16 oz almond milk

⅛ cup plus 1 tbsp **pure birch xylitol** (SmartSweet brand is my choice)

2 tsp non-GMO **lecithin powder**

1 ½ tsp **yacon powder**

1 tsp **tocotrienols powder**

1 ½ tsp **mesquite pod meal** powder

½ tsp **mucuna prureins** powder

7 scoops **stevia** (if your stevia comes with a small scoop)

A pinch or two of **Celtic** or **Himalayan** salt to taste

14 ice cubes

Place all ingredients in blender, adding ice cubes last. If you do not have a high power blender, add the ice cubes slowly. Blend and enjoy.

This is Green Smoothie Challenge approved. Feel free to ingest 6 – 8 ounces of these treats every couple of days. You will not know this is not a real chocolate milkshake. It is amazing!

The above shake contains a few ingredients that may be unfamiliar to you. These are known as superfoods and I have gone into detail about each in Chapter 2. The initial purchase of such ingredients may require a small investment. Consider it a deposit into your health savings account. These ingredients will last quite some time. You will not be replacing them often so in the long run it's a small price to pay for something you will enjoy over, and over. Offering a taste of this shake to people is the number one way I introduce others to the world of living and high nutrition foods.

Rippo Family Soda Pop

1 bottle mineral water

2 limes

6 scoops of stevia

Pour mineral water into a pretty pitcher. Squeeze juice from limes. Mix ingredients together and enjoy over ice.

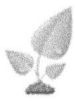

Maria's Hunger Eliminator Shake

20 oz almond milk

1 ½ tbsp maca

⅛ tsp ashwagandha extract powder

⅛ tsp macuna pruriens powder

1 ½ tsp yacon root powder

1 ½ tsp mesquite powder

½ tsp raw tocotrienols

⅛ tsp salt, Celtic or Himalayan

½ tsp vanilla

3 scoops stevia

¼ cup pure birch xylitol or sweetener of choice, i.e. raw honey

½ tsp cinnamon

¼ tsp nutmeg

Place all ingredients in the blender and blend well. Foam will form on top for you to use to make a latte. The drink may be warmed in your blender or on the stovetop. Do not heat above 118° F in order to preserve the enzymes and nutrients! Alternatively, you may replace some of the almond milk with ice cubes and make a frozen shake. Simply add about 10 – 12 large-ish ice cubes and blend until desired consistency is reached.

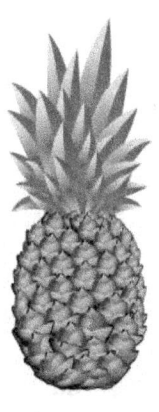

CHAPTER 7
After The Challenge

Coming Off of The Challenge

> *Even a fool can fast, but only a wise man knows how to break the fast properly and to build up properly after the fast. – Dr. Otto Buchinger, author of The Therapuetic Fasting Cure*

Now that you have not been eating your normal diet for a time and your body has been cleansing, it is of utmost importance that you *slowly* begin adding foods back into your diet. You may feel tempted to eat a lot, but this can be very damaging to your system. Your body has had a break from producing the enzymes normally used to digest the food you eat. Adding foods back in slowly gives your body the ability to adjust enzyme production and prepare for the hard work of digestion again. Take at least four days to reintroduce whole foods to your diet. Soups and salads along with fermented dairy products such as yogurt and kefir are a good place to start. Make delightful salad dressings to please your palate. Continue drinking your smoothies and listen to your body to see what foods work well for you. I have included some delectable raw dishes at the end of this book. Experiment with those after three or four days of reintroducing foods. Eat slowly and chew your food very well. Raw nuts and seeds are an excellent choice for snacks, but if you have avoided them on the Challenge, wait until the fourth day to reintroduce them. Eat avocados and other fresh fruits and veggies. If you choose to add dairy and meat products back into your diet, consider choosing raw milk cheeses and free range, organic meats. Add these back in slowly and start by eating meat boiled in soup with broth and plenty of vegetables.

A Healthy Diet After The Challenge

A longevity diet is a lifestyle that promotes healing and slows the aging process. There is no magic pill to take. There is not one diet that works for every person. I can find an expert for every imaginable diet that will convince you, using scientific evidence, that their diet is **the one** that works. Each individual is unique in their genetic make-up. What works for one person may make another sick. Most diets *do* work for some people. I know people who have been cured of diseases on a 100% raw-food diet and I know of others who became ill on the same diet. I have met healthy vegetarians and sickly ones. The same is true for those who eat animal products. It is important to know your metabolic type to determine if you require high protein, high carbohydrates or a mixture of both. Dr. Mercola has an amazing resource on his Web site at **www.mercola.com**. It is a free Nutritional Typing test. I highly recommend finding out your type and then designing *your* optimal diet around this. If you wish to follow a strictly raw-food diet, Dr. Gabriel Cousens teaches you how to customize your diet by determining your metabolic bio-individuality in his book **Conscious Eating**. I also offer metabolic typing. **Visit http://www.mariarippo.com/book-an-appointment.html** to book an appointment with me.

A diet for a long, healthy life consists of balanced nutrition, good sleep, exercise, slowing and deepening your breath, hydration, mental and spiritual health as well as knowing what your purpose is and working towards your dream. This may seem impossible to some, but working towards balance in these areas (while accepting the inevitability of lack of balance) will bring about true health. I have touched on many of these areas already. Here I am going to focus a bit more on what makes up a healthy diet.

It is made up largely of fresh, organic fruits and vegetables, nuts and seeds, sea vegetables, cultured foods, raw dairy products, whole grains and white rice for some people along with quality animal products and plenty of healthy fat. Many people are opposed to eating animal products. It is important to remain open to the idea of eating high quality, pasture raised animal products if you are not doing well on a raw-food, vegan or vegetarian diet. There are certain nutrients that you simply do not get if eating a purely vegan diet. The one that all health experts agree on is Vitamin B-12, which only comes from animal products. The list of healthy foods above may seem rather limiting at first glance but I have included an amazing recipe section that will enable you to make delicious foods from the vibrant living foods mentioned above. Visit your local farmer's market just to see how many beautiful choices there are when it comes to fresh fruits and vegetables. There are many possibilities!

Along with these nutritious foods, I feel it is important to include the fat-soluble activators A, D, E and K, which come from animal fats such as organ meats, butter fats, egg yolks and sea food. Bone broth, raw milk and fermented cod liver oil are worthy of consideration as well. Most of these foods are best in their raw form excluding bone broth. Butter and organ meats from grazing animals and some seafood are good sources of what Weston A. Price referred to as *Activator X*. These foods give your body the ability to drive minerals into your bones and assimilate the nutrients you eat. These healthy fats will help you feel satisfied with less unhealthy food cravings. You can find out more about these healing foods through the Weston A. Price Foundation at **www.westonaprice.org**. Most importantly, learn how to properly prepare these foods so they nourish your body. I also find much wisdom in the Ayurvedic way of life. Two helpful books to learn more are Deepak Chopra's, *Perfect Health* and Madhuri Phillips book *Your Irresistible Life*.

Another very important ingredient to consider is calorie restriction (which is very simple with a whole food lifestyle). The more we eat, the more enzymes stores we use up and the more energy it takes for our body to digest. Digestion is the number energy zapper. It is a major factor in aging as well!

My one eating rule is to only eat when I am good and hungry and to stop when I am satisfied; not uncomfortably stuffed full, but no longer hungry. Learn to feel how food makes you feel instead of obsessing over numbers of calories or fat grams. Trust your body to tell you when it's had enough and make sure to eat healthy treats here and there. What calorie restriction does not mean is that you eat so little that you are not feeding your body enough calories.

A good rule to follow is eat breakfast like a king, lunch like a queen and dinner like a pauper. It is wise not to snack between meals. Allow your body to become hungry, good and hungry, before you eat again after your last meal. Following these guidelines eliminates any need to count calories or fat grams!

In one study on caloric restrictions conducted in 2004, it was found that "caloric restriction acts rapidly, even in old mice, to extend remaining lifespan by 42% and to dramatically reduce tumors as a cause of death." The findings of the study also suggested that "gene expression also changes rapidly to a new pattern that is closely associated with lower cancer mortality and better health." The easiest way I have found to do this is simply to eat when you are very hungry and stop when you are satisfied, when you are no longer hungry, but not stuffed full. Go to bed more on the hungry side, not so hungry that you can't fall asleep, but a bit hungry. Since digestion takes so much energy, you don't want to be doing it while you are attempting to rest and rejuvenate as

---

[63] Spindler, Stephen R, PhD, 'Reversing Aging Rapidly with Short-term Calorie Restriction', Life Extension Magazine, 2007.

it can greatly diminish your health and energy levels. Stop eating three hours before going to bed. This will allow your body to repair and rest while you sleep and you will wake up feeling much more rested. It is important to allow our bodies to repair at night. If your body is spending the first four hours of the night digesting food instead of making necessary repairs, chances are you will be sick more often, experience more disease and take years off your life. Our bodies do their physical repair work from 10 p.m. until 2 a.m. and their psychological repair work from 2 a.m. until 6 a.m. If we do not sleep during these hours, we are not giving our body's adequate time to repair. Lack of sleep causes stress levels to rise, which in turn causes sugar and caffeine cravings. This leads to weight gain and fat storage as well as hormonal imbalance. What a simple thing you can do: go to bed a bit hungry to live longer and stay thinner! If night eating is an issue for you, visit my website at **www.mariarippo.com** and go to the 'free downloads' tab where you find a lot of help for working through your cravings.

Did you know that what you don't eat is more important than what you do eat? Yes there are some foods that are so destructive to our health that we should just stay away from them altogether. And some foods are so healthy for us that we should include them in our diets every day. For many people, the idea of giving up certain foods is so overwhelming that they do not even want to attempt to become healthy. Well, I propose a new way of thinking about how to get healthy. Forget trying to give up anything! We have so many emotional connections to food that the idea of giving them up permanently simply seems impossible. So, consider not trying to give anything up! Instead, add some **healthy foods** to your daily diet. The more healthy things you commit to eating on a daily basis and the less you try to restrict yourself, the more you will begin to desire the healthy foods and not crave the damaging foods.

Take it step by step. Add a new, healthy food to your diet each month. For example, start with fermented or cultured foods one month, add green juices the next, add good fats such as raw butter and cod liver oil (or **fermented cod liver oil and high vitamin butter oil from www.greenpasture.org**, my all-time favorite daily supplement!) or coconut oil another month, etc. Eat with the seasons and be sure to rotate your food choices. This is easier when you eat what is in season, as you will naturally rotate your diet throughout the year. Eating the same foods over, and over can cause food sensitivities. I became sensitive to berries after putting them in my smoothies every day for two years. I can eat them now in small amounts, but I had to take a break from them for a year or so.

If you find that you are comforting yourself with food, simply admit it and try to find other ways to feel comforted. Find your passion in life and go after it. Work on forgiving yourself and those you love. Get rid of bitterness towards yourself and others, especially those close to you. Find your way to your loveliness that has been hidden down somewhere inside of you waiting to be acknowledged. You have value. You are precious. Love the person you were made to be. Feel your feelings instead of overeating in order to ignore them. It can seem scary to become aware of your emotions but at the end of the day, after having cried, screamed, kicked or heaved, you will see that you are still alive, in fact, much more alive. When a person chooses to fight the obsession and pretend it does not exist, it only beckons more intensely for our attention. When we stop trying to change the unchangeable and accept what is and begin to be grateful for all parts of our lives and to see our own loveliness, then everything will change. Improving emotional wellbeing is an essential ingredient for optimal health. Stress is the worst offender of good health!

The foods that are number one on the list of foods to avoid are refined sugars and processed carbohydrates. These are the most damaging to the system. If you decide not to avoid anything else, adding lots of greens and raw foods as well as cultured vegetables and bone broth and avoiding the foods above will make a big difference in your health. The other foods to avoid are table salt, white flour and pasteurized dairy. You can make an amazing improvement to your health by taking these slowly out of your diet and replacing them with healthier alternatives.

My Top Twelve Tips for Health and Vitality

1. If, at all possible, stop eating refined sugars and processed carbohydrates. Instead, choose sprouted grain breads such as Ezekiel 4:9 brand, whole grain flours and natural sweeteners such as raw honey, dates and stevia. Work towards eating fewer grains and focus on quinoa, millet, amaranth and buckwheat, as these are much easier to digest than wheat, rye, barley, etc. I prefer to use coconut flour and almond flour for baking. Check out **www.elanaspantry.com** for recipes. Also check out my website at **www.mariarippo.com** for my favorites!

2. Eat a big salad full of dark greens and lots of colorful vegetables (or a lightly steamed mixture of veggies) every single day. Use a natural dressing or make one with olive oil, raw apple cider vinegar, Celtic salt and fresh cracked pepper. For an extra boost, chop up some fresh garlic and use fresh herbs or mustard and some **stevia** for sweetening. See Maria's Honey Mustard Vinaigrette in the recipe section. Check out my 'Dressings' at **www.mariarippo.com**

3. Decide to eat sweet things every day if you crave sweets but with this one condition—use nourishing ingredients such as whole grain flour, natural sweeteners and healthy fats. Check out this book for good ideas: *The Raw Food Detox Diet*, by Natalia Rose or *Nourishing Traditions*, by Sally Fallon. There are so many amazing ice creams, cookies, brownies, etc. that you can make with carefully selected, nutritious ingredients so that they are actually adding to your health instead of taking away from it. Many of these have a lot of good fat in

them which will actually help your body rid itself of fat. Healthy fats are a key to weight loss because they help you feel satiated and keep the food craving monsters at bay while nourishing the 'happy center' of the brain. Healthy fats include raw milk cream, pasture butter (from grass-fed dairy cows), coconut oil, cod liver oil, raw or lightly cooked egg yolks from pastured chickens, extra virgin olive oil, flax oil, nuts and seeds.

4. Add **bone broth** to your diet along with added **gelatin**.

5. Get your sleep and exercise. These are both vital to your well-being. Turn off your TV. I have never heard a hard-working, successful person say, "Boy, I am sure glad I spent time watching TV every day. It really helped me succeed." Get an inspiring book to read before you go to sleep or get out into nature instead.

6. Add some sea vegetables to your diet such as Nori, Dulse and Wakame. You can simply buy some Dulse and add it to your salad dressing or just sprinkle it on your food. Sea vegetables are very high in vitamins, minerals and even trace minerals. Take digestive enzymes with each meal.

7. Drink more **pure water**. Water does an amazing job of detoxifying and hydrating your body. The trick though is to not drink water with your meals. This will dilute your digestive juices and cause your body to not be able to digest efficiently. Wait at least one hour after a meal and do not drink anything thirty minutes before you eat. It is amazing how much energy you will get from doing this. Also, sometimes thirst is disguised as hunger. So there is a good chance that when you drink water, that hungry feeling will go away. For extra hydration, add some **Crystal Energy**® or **Megahydrate**™ to each glass of water you drink. This will give your cells extra hydration, giving you more energy and vitality. First thing in the morning, add the juice of ½ of a fresh lemon to your water. For extra cleansing, add 1 tablespoon of raw apple cider vinegar plus ⅛ teaspoon Celtic or Himalayan salt to 25+ ounces of water to consume during your day.

8. Try to make the switch from coffee to green tea, white tea or even better, a non-caffeinated herbal tea if possible. Drinking tea at the end of a meal is a good way to get your mind off of food and onto something that is a great ritual, but will not add calories.

9. If you feel the desire to eat, but you ate within two hours, you may actually be looking for a way to change your mood. See if you can find something to occupy yourself for at least one hour. Set a timer and drink some water. Tell yourself that you will eat in one hour. This will set your mind at ease. Then find a way to stay occupied or a way to feel fulfilled for that hour.

10. Work on your thought life and your self-talk. Begin to take notice of the things you regularly tell yourself. Are your first thoughts in the morning ones of gratitude or of complaint? Actively begin to think more positively. Think of three things you are thankful for the minute you wake up. Think of three reasons you are happy to be you. Your circumstances may be beyond your control, but your thoughts and behaviors are yours to choose.

11. Consume **kefir** and other **fermented foods**. These amazing immune-enhancing, health-building foods will put your body in balance and fight disease. You can find instructions for making kefir out of fresh almond and other nut milks in Gabriel Cousens book, ***Rainbow Green Live-Food Cuisine***. Also, ***The Body Ecology Diet***, by Donna Gates is an amazing resource for making cultured foods and eating a healthy diet as in ***The Gaps Diet***. One reason I love cultured vegetables is they taste so good and last a long time. I don't have to worry about them going bad.

12. Eat gluten free and for a time, remove grains from your diet to see how you feel.

How to Make Your Own Cultured/Fermented Foods

Cultured vegetables have a long history dating back to the Ancient Chinese, the Romans and even Genghis Khan's army. It is what was consumed by Dutch seamen and found to prevent scurvy. Sauerkraut, German for "sour cabbage," is the most familiar form of cultured vegetables although most commercial varieties of sauerkraut are pasteurized and do not contain the necessary healthy bacteria that make this food so healing and health building. There are raw versions of cultured foods available in health food stores and online. Fermented vegetables are teeming with the healthy bacteria known as lactobacillus. These bacteria enter into the digestive tract when the cultured food is consumed. Eating or drinking cultured **foods and beverages** is the most natural and effective way to get many enzymes and good bacteria into the intestines. This is a very important part of any optimal **health program** and a much less expensive alternative to purchasing costly probiotics and enzyme supplements.

Cultured vegetables include foods like sauerkraut, kimchi, tsukemono, and cultured pickles. Fermented **beverages** include drinks like kefir and kambucha. Cultured vegetables are a great way to add raw vegetables to the diet when uncultured raw vegetables are too difficult to digest. Cultured vegetables benefit digestive health greatly and heal **candida** because they are able to balance the good-to-bad bacteria ratio in the intestines. This is especially important in today's society because it is estimated that up to 90% of the world population is unknowingly suffering from candida. Candida is the overgrowth of yeast in the intestines and can spread to all major organs in the body. It can go undetected by conventional doctors and over time wreaks havoc on a person's health.

Sauerkraut is made from shredded cabbage, placed in an airtight container with a vegetable culture starter, and left to sit out at room temperature for three to seven days while the healthy bacteria go to work. It is then refrigerated and can last up eight to twelve months if kept cool.

Cultured vegetables contain lactobacilli (friendly bacteria) which create an environment where candida does not thrive. They have also been found effective in treating "peptic ulcers, ulcerative colitis, colic, food allergies, cystitis and constipation." Cultured vegetables have also been used in the treatment and prevention of cancer.

Another major benefit of cultured foods is their high content of **enzymes**. Oftentimes, natural health experts will say that good bacteria and enzymes are the key to disease prevention and longevity. Consuming live enzymes with every meal will have an amazingly positive affect on overall health and longevity. Because of the live enzymes content, fermented vegetables aid in the digestion of all foods they are eaten with, especially starches and proteins. They also improve the absorption of the nutrients from any accompanying foods.

According to Viktoras Kulvinskus, co-founder of the Hippocrates Health Institute and author of *Survival into the 21st Century* and other books, consuming cultured vegetables is one way to prevent sicknesses such as the swine flu. A helpful guide to fermenting your foods very inexpensively is **Wild Fermentation**, by Sandor Katz.

If you prefer to purchase cultured vegetables, you will find them in their raw form for sale in most health food grocery stores. If they are pastuerized, they will not contain the health enhancing properties. If you'd like to try making your own, my friend Kael Nielson, a certified body ecologist, has been kind enough to share her recipes below.

---

[64] Cousens, Gabriel, MD, *Rainbow Green Live-Food Cuisine,* North Atlantic books, Berkeley, CA, 2003.

[65] Kulvinskus Viktoras, Interview with Kevin Gianni

Green Blend

1 green cabbage

1 white or yellow onion

1 celery, bunch

1 head garlic, whole

2 kale, bunches

2 inches gingerroot, peeled

1 tbsp Celtic or Himalayan salt, per pound of veggies

Supplies:

stainless steel, glass or ceramic containers, with air-tight seals

knife, vegetable peeler and cutting board

food processor (optional)

large mixing bowl and spoon

Steps:

1. Wash all vegetables well, and remove outer leaves of cabbage for later use.

2. Chop, slice or grate vegetables (by hand or with food processor) and combine in a large bowl.

3. Add salt and knead vegetables for 3 – 5 minutes.

4. Pack vegetables tightly into chosen containers, using a spoon or potato masher. Leave at least 2 inches at top of jar for expansion. Add water if necessary to bring the liquid level above the top of the veggies.

5. Wash outer leaves of cabbage, roll them up and place over top of the packed veggies to keep veggies submerged under water.

6. Secure lid tightly (Fermentation is an anaerobic process, so it is important to protect the product from contact with air.)

7. Leave to culture at room temperature (between 70° and 80° F) in a darkened corner.

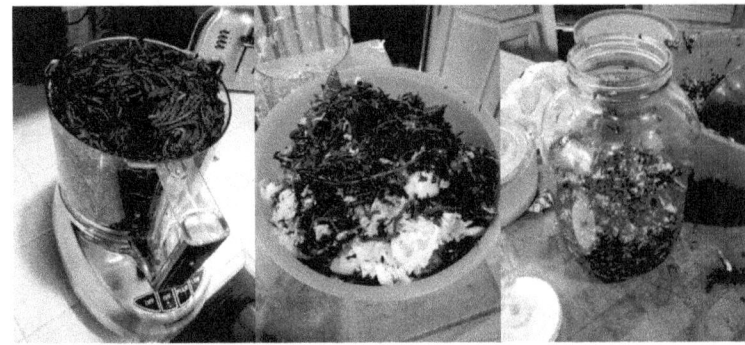

8. Culture the vegetables a minimum 3-7 days or up to several months. Some say cultured vegetables are like fine wine – they improve with age.

9. Once opened and exposed to air, they must be kept in the refrigerator. This will slow down the culturing process but not stop it completely. A layer of harmless mold may form on top of the cabbage leaves; simply scoop off and discard so as not to affect the flavor of the veggies. Since pathogenic bacteria, which spoil food, will not be able to take over in the presence of so many friendly bacteria, the vegetables will keep many months in the refrigerator.

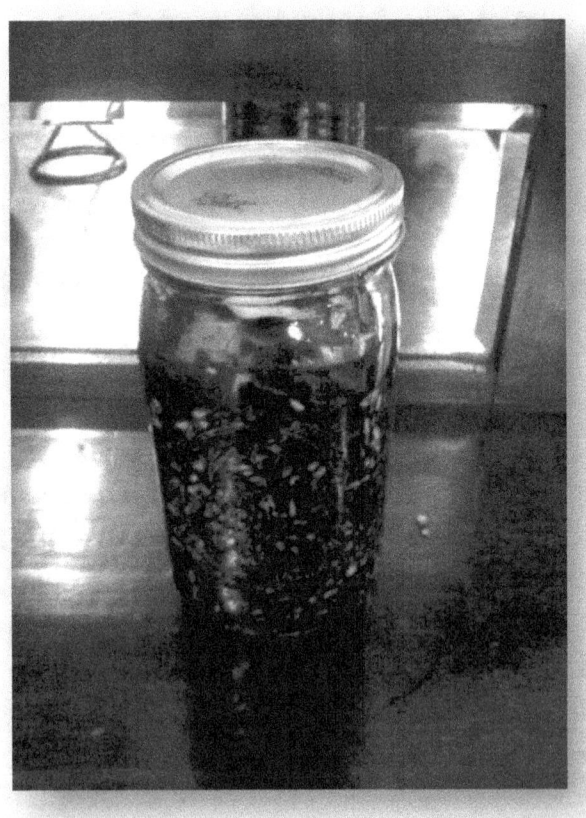

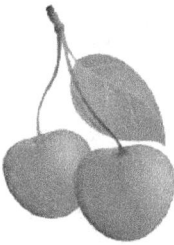

CHAPTER 8
Raw Food Recipes to Warm Your Heart and Fatten Your Soul

The best time to prepare some yummy, raw foods for you and your family is right after taking The Challenge. Your sense of taste is heightened and these healthy foods will taste amazing. It is a perfect time to introduce foods that are very high in nutrition to your taste buds, emotions and body and, at the same time, very satisfying and delicious. When eating these foods, instead of processed and refined foods, you will be able to experience the same kind of energy, vitality and mental clarity that being on The Green Smoothie Challenge gives you.

Appetizers

Almond Seed Crackers

I regularly bring these to parties on an appetizer plate with my guacamole, almond ricotta dip and veggie sticks. Gabriel Cousens, MD, has lovingly shared this recipe.

This recipe is my family's favorite raw cracker recipe. You can find this recipe along with many other health transforming, delectable raw food recipes in his book *Rainbow Green Live-Food Cuisine*. Sir Gabriel Cousens MD, MD(H), DD, founder and director of the Tree of Life Rejuvenation Center, is a leading author, and world expert in raw, living foods nutrition. You will find more about his work and the Tree of Life Center at **www.treeoflife.nu**.

6 cups flax seed, soaked for 8 hours in pure water

4 cups almonds soaked 12 hours in pure water

4 cups carrot pulp

2 cups parsley, finely chopped

1 cup sesame seeds, soaked 4 hours

1 cup pumpkin seeds, soaked 4 hours

6 celery stalks, finely chopped

6 tbsp lemon juice, fresh *(I prefer to use only 3 tbsp)*

3 tbsp Celtic sea salt *(I prefer to use 1 tbsp, taste, then add more if desired)*

3 tbsp kelp, powdered *(I prefer to use Dulse, which can be easier to find in any health food or Asian market)*

Drain and rinse all nuts and seeds. Process almonds and carrots in a Champion® juicer with the solid plate or in a food processor.

Combine all ingredients in a large mixing bowl and mix well. *I personally prefer to mix all ingredients in a food processor.*

Spread the dough on a dehydrator* tray with a non-stick sheet or oiled parchment paper approximately ¼" thick. If using parchment paper, rub with olive oil before spreading dough to prevent sticking.

Score crackers with a spatula or pizza cutter. Dehydrate at 145° F for the first 2 – 3 hours, then turn over, remove dehydrator sheet and continue dehydrating at 115° F for 6 – 8 hours or until desired moisture is obtained.

Store in glass container. Makes nine 14"-by-14" trays.

*If you do not own a dehydrator, use cookie sheets and place them in your oven on the lowest setting with the oven door cracked open.

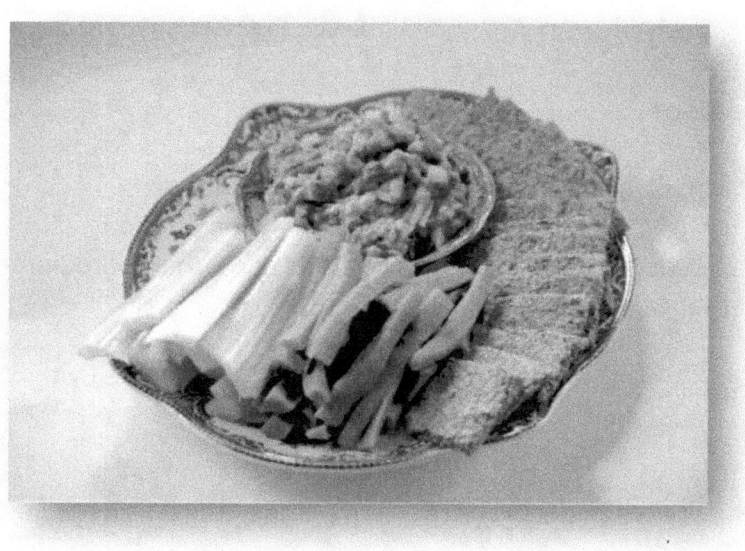

Maria's Guacamole

1 avocado

1 tbsp onion, minced

1 small garlic clove

1 tbsp tomato, minced

2 tsp lemon juice, fresh squeezed

1 tbsp cilantro, chopped

Celtic sea salt or Himalayan salt to taste

Scoop flesh out of avocado skins. Place in bowl and add other ingredients. Mash ingredients together using a fork. Enjoy!

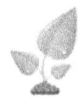

Maria's Almond "Ricotta" Dip

1 cup raw almonds (soaked overnight)

⅓ of an onion

⅛ cup olive oil

⅛ cup raw almond butter

juice of 1 lemon

Celtic or Himalayan salt to taste.

Drain and rinse almonds. Place all ingredients in food processor and process until it becomes a smooth, dip-like consistency. Making this one day ahead will give the flavors time to meld together and become very rich.

Serve with raw crackers and veggies such as celery, cucumber, carrot, cauliflower, jicama and red bell pepper. This is great to take to a party and everyone will enjoy it!

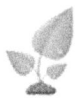

Maria's Nacho Cheez Dip

1 cup soaked almonds

1 red bell pepper

1 jalapeno, deseeded

1 clove garlic, minced

juice of 1 lemon

3 tbsp nutritional yeast

⅛ onion, chopped

1 tsp salt

Drain and rinse nuts. Mix all ingredients in food processor and serve with cut up veggies or flax crackers. You may also spread this mixture on a dehydrated tray lined with a Teflex sheet and dry it to make 'slices' of cheez.

Maria's Festive Seed Cheez

1 cup almond pulp from making almond milk, hung in sprout bag over night

⅛ cup sundried tomatoes, chopped, soaked in olive oil

6 dried olives, chopped

1 tbsp lemon juice

½ tsp salt

3 scoops stevia

1 clove garlic, minced

¼ cup parsley, chopped

2 tbsp olive oil from soaking tomatoes

Combine all ingredients in bowl until well blended. Form into a cheez ball and serve with crackers and veggie sticks on a beautiful platter! Great to use on raw pizza with your favorite veggie toppings.

Maria's Sprouted Sun-Dried Tomato Hummus

½ cup sundried tomatoes, soaked in 2 tbsp olive oil over night

1 ½ cups garbanzo beans: *soak raw beans overnight, rinse and drain. Place in colander and cover with pot lid. Rinse twice in 24 hours to sprout the beans. Rinse well before using.*

1 – 2 garlic cloves, minced

2 tbsp lemon juice

1 tbsp tahini

1 tsp cumin

½ tsp grated lemon zest

½ tsp Celtic or Himalayan salt

Place ingredients in food processor and mix well. Serve with raw crackers and veggie sticks.

Snacks

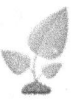

Maria's Un-Roasted Pumpkin Pie Nuts

My kids beg me for these!

2 tbsp Xylitol or Agave Nectar

3 scoops stevia

2 tsp vanilla

Liberal amount of Himalayan salt

2 heaping tsp pumpkin pie spice

2 cups nuts of choice, soaked overnight, drained and rinsed; *walnuts are great*

Place all ingredients into a bowl with the nuts to marinate. Let this sit for 2 hours. Place on non-stick sheet or parchment paper in dehydrator or on a cookie sheet in oven on lowest setting with the oven door left open. Dehydrate until crisp and roasted-like.

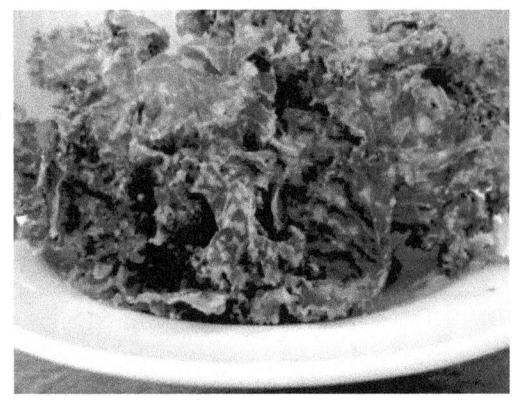

Maria's Cheezy Un-Potato Chips (Kale Chips)

2 large bunches of curly kale, rinsed, deveined; break into chip-size pieces

2 lemons

2 red bell peppers

1 ⅛ cups raw cashews, soaked 4 – 6 hours

Himalayan or Celtic salt to taste

5 tbsp nutritional yeast

Chop the red pepper into small pieces; add to a blender or food processor with lemon juice. Blend until smooth. Add the cashews, cayenne pepper and ⅛ teaspoon salt and again blend until smooth. Next add the nutritional yeast and blend again. *Blending in stages gives you the smooth texture you will need.*

Place kale in one or two large bowls and pour marinade over it. Massage the kale leaves with the marinade and let sit for about 15 minutes. Next, place kale pieces on dehydrator trays lined with non-stick sheets or parchment paper and dehydrate at 115° F. After 2 hours, remove the kale chips from parchment paper or non-stick sheets and place directly on mesh dehydrator sheets.

By the time they have been drying for eight hours, they should be seriously crunchy. If they aren't, just leave them in until they are!

Taste, and if they're not salty enough, sprinkle some over and then munch, munch, munch! If you do not own a dehydrator, simple do the steps above using cookie sheets and the lowest setting you can set your oven on. Keep the oven door open.

Salads

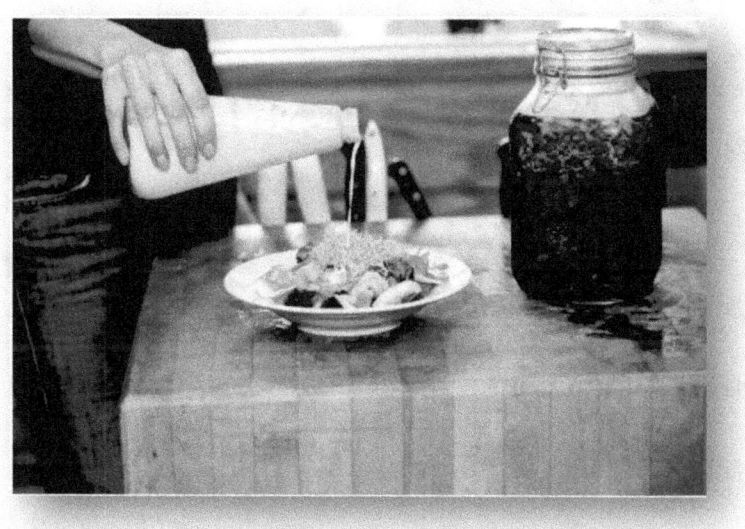

Maria's Favorite "Blue Cheez" Salad Dressing

1 cup raw sesame tahini

¾ cup pure water

⅛ cup fresh basil

⅛ cup fresh parsley

⅓ cup fresh lemon juice

1 tbsp fresh oregano

1 tsp Himalayan or Celtic salt

1 tbsp Dulse (seaweed)

Combine all ingredients in blender and mix until smooth. Enjoy on your daily salad.

Maria's 'Honey' Mustard Vinaigrette

2 parts olive oil

1 part raw, unpasteurized apple cider vinegar

1 tbsp mustard

2 tiny scoops of stevia *(the stevia usually comes with a scooper in it)*

sea salt or Himalayan salt, to taste

Fresh ground pepper, to taste

1 – 2 cloves fresh garlic, finely minced

Place all ingredients in a beautiful dressing jar. Shake like there's no tomorrow! Enjoy.

Maria's Sprouted Wheat Salad

3 cups sprouted red winter wheat: *Soak sprouting wheat berries for 6 hours in pure water. Drain and rinse. Place in colander and cover with a pot lid. Rinse and drain twice a day for 5 days keeping covered between rinses. Now they are ready to use.*

½ cup chopped green onions

¼ cup chopped parsley

⅜ tsp dry mustard

2 tbsp minced garlic

¼ cup raw apple cider vinegar

⅛ cup of lemon juice

¼ tsp salt

Dash of cayenne pepper

⅛ tsp agave nectar

½ red bell pepper, chopped

½ cup olive oil

Mix all ingredients together and let stand for 1 hour to marinate. Serve as a side dish or on top of a green salad as a meal.

Soups

My friend, Maya Deva Adjani (a.k.a Maya Papaya) has graciously shared these soup recipes. Maya is a raw food chef, educator and the creator of Breathe Eat Dance Evolve. You may find out more about Maya's work at **www.BreatheEatDanceEvolve.com**.

Curry Ginger Soup

Equipment

food processor

The Base

4 carrots

3 tbsp coconut butter

2 cloves garlic

2 inches fresh ginger

¾ inches fresh turmeric root

Juice of 1 lime

2 tbsp raw tahini

1 tbsp curry powder

1 avocado, peeled and pitted

juice of 1 orange

pinch of cayenne

salt or Nama Shoyu, to taste

For Serving

1 avocado, pitted and sliced into cubes

1 cucumber, peeled and cubed

cherry tomatoes

½ Fuji apple, chopped

Prepare

Place base ingredients in food processor and blend until desired consistency is reached. Add water or lime juice, as needed to blend. Place avocado, cucumber, cherry tomato and apple in serving in bowls; pour soup on top. Garnish with fresh parsley and green onion.

Raw Winter Squash Soup

<u>The Base</u>

4 cups yellow squash

4 cups fresh-squeezed orange juice

2 ripe avocados, peeled and pitted

6 dates, pitted

⅛ jalapeño pepper

2 tbsp raw coconut butter

1 tbsp Nama Shoyu (raw soy sauce)

3+ tsp curry powder

⅛ tsp cumin

2 inches of ginger

2 cloves garlic

<u>Prepare</u>

Place all ingredients in blender, adding water as needed, and blend until creamy.

Pour into serving bowls with chopped onion, parsley, tomato and apple or pear. Garnish with dill and parsley.

<u>For Serving</u>

add parsley, finely chopped

1 tomato, cubed

1 apple or pear, cubed

1 green onion, chopped

Sustenance

Nori Burritos

Simply use untoasted sheets of Nori as your tortilla and fill with seed cheez, avocado or hummus, along with all of your favorite veggies such as sprouts, lettuce, tomato, cucumber, cabbage, etc. You can even add some mustard, olives or both!

The Sun Kitchen Cheezburgers

This recipe is shared courtesy of Bruce Horowitz, author of *The Sun Kitchen Un-Cook Book*. Bruce is the former executive chef of the world's first live-food restaurant, Raw, in San Francisco. He has served as the executive chef at the world's largest live-food gathering, Raw Spirit Festival in 2007 and 2008. To find out more about Bruce's work, his permaculture design business or his raw chef certification program visit **www.thesunkitchen.com**.

Tip: For 'char-broiled' burgers, baste with flax oil.

1 ½ cups each walnuts and sunflower seeds, soaked for four hours and rinsed

½ cup chopped onion

½ cup chopped celery

½ cup chopped sweet pepper

½ cup sundried tomato pieces (or 1 cup cherry tomato halves)

¼ – ½ cup any of the following herbs: rosemary, parsley, basil, dill, oregano or thyme

3 tbsp Nama Shoyu soy sauce, miso or 2 tbsp sea salt

2 tbsp olive oil

2 – 4 garlic cloves

1 – 3 rounded tsp ground cumin

"heat" to taste (such as cayenne pepper)

Place walnuts, sunflower seeds, garlic, herbs, onion, celery and pepper through juicer with blank. You may alternatively use a food processor. Mix in salt, 'heat', oil, cumin and sundried tomatoes. Form into burgers and dehydrate for 3 – 6 hours at 105° F.

Serve with Alissa Cohen's burger buns, Maria's nacho cheez dip, avocado, lettuce, tomato, pickles and whatever else tantalizes your taste buds!

Alissa Cohen's Burger Buns

Alissa Cohen, author of *Living on Live Food,* has generously shared this recipe. An internationally recognized author, speaker, raw food chef and consultant, Alissa's devoted following includes thousands of people throughout the world who have maintained successful weight losses, healed themselves of a myriad of diseases, and swear by her simple and fun approach to fantastic health. Learn more about Alissa and her work or get her book at **www.alissacohen.com**.

These look and taste like real burger buns if you shape them round and full and sprinkle them with sesame seeds. You can also make bread, crackers and pizza crust out of this dough. The thinner you roll out the dough (as you would for crackers or pizza) the faster it will dehydrate.

2 cups sprouted buckwheat

⅜ cups soaked whole flax seeds

⅜ cup carrots

⅛ cup olive oil

1 tsp curry

1 tsp fresh rosemary (or ⅛ tsp dried)

1 tsp fresh thyme (or ⅛ tsp dried)

1 clove garlic

1 tsp salt

sesame seeds (optional)

Grind the carrots in a food processor until they are diced. Add other ingredients and blend well until dough-like. Form into buns and place on mesh screens on dehydrator screens. Sprinkle with sesame seeds, if desired. Dehydrate at 105° F for 24 hours.

The Sun Kitchen Perfect Pesto

Another great recipe contributed by Bruce Horowitz of The Sun Kitchen **www.thesunkitchen.com**. Thank you, Bruce!

2 cups walnuts

2 bunches basil, mostly de-stemmed

2 – 6 cloves garlic

½ tsp sea salt or to taste

Process all ingredients. Add water, olive oil and a spritz of lemon juice, if desired. The mixture should clump together when done. Do not over-process.

Mama Maria's Italian Pizza Crust

2 ½ cups sprouted buckwheat: *soak 1 ½ cups of organic buckwheat sprouting grouts in pure water for one hour. Place in colander and rinse very well. Place colander over a pot then place pot lid over colander. Rinse the buckwheat very well about four times in 24 – 36 hours. When you see a "tail" it is ready.*

4 carrots, chopped

1 cup ground flax seeds

¼ cup olive oil

1 ½ tsp Celtic or Himalayan salt

1 tbsp Italian seasonings

Place sprouted buckwheat in food processor and mix. Slowly add ¼ cup olive oil. Process until a ball of dough is formed. Place aside in bowl. Add chopped carrots to processor and process. Add the rest of the ingredients to carrot mixture in processor and mix well. Place all ingredients in bowl and "knead."

Form three balls of dough. Place each ball on a non-stick dehydrator sheet or oiled parchment paper on dehydrator tray. Dehydrate at 145° F for 2 hours. Turn dehydrator down to 115° and continue dehydrating to desired texture, about 8 hours.

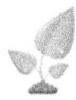

Kevin and Annmarie Gianni's Meatless Meatballs

This recipe is shared by Kevin and Annmarie Gianni. They are the hosts of the daily Internet show, The Renegade Health Show. Kevin is a health advocate, author, interviewer and film consultant. Annmarie has been involved in athletics and healthy living since childhood. She received her Sports Medicine degree from East Carolina University. To get their books and learn more about them, or to download a free copy of Kevin's book, High Raw, visit **www.renegadehealth.com**. Kevin's research is what finally helped me see that my raw vegan diet was causing a lot of deficiencies.

1 cup of soaked walnuts

1 ½ cups cremini or portabella mushrooms, coarsely chopped

olive oil

Nama Shoyu soy sauce

4 cloves garlic

thyme

oregano

parsley

Italian seasoning

crushed red pepper

flax seed oil

sea salt to taste

Marinate walnuts and mushrooms at least 1 hour with a little Nama Shoyu, olive oil and 2 cloves garlic. In a food processor, blend together with 2 more cloves garlic, thyme, oregano, parsley, crushed red pepper, flax seed oil or olive oil, sea salt to taste. We always end up adding a bit more Italian season mix. Form balls using about 1 ½ tbsp of mixture at a time, and dehydrate for 4 to 6 hours at 115° F.

Serve the above recipe with marinara sauce from *Rainbow Green Live-Food Cuisine*, by Gabriel Cousens or *Living on Live Food*, by Alissa Cohen. A great topping is a product called 'Rawmesan' which you can find at a health food store or raw food store.

Treats

Angela Stokes-Monarch's Truffles

Angela lost an amazing 160 lbs. with a raw lifestyle, reversing morbid obesity. Her book, *Raw Emotions* explores raw transformations beyond the physical level.

Sweet raw truffles can easily be made up in batches and kept in the fridge or freezer for instant sweet satisfaction as desired. Here is a basic sample recipe to start with:

3–5 tbsp (to taste) of powdered sweetener of your choice – e.g. lucuma, yacon, mesquite powders (*not* stevia in these quantities)

3 tbsp almond butter OR 1 cup soaked nuts of your choice, e.g. walnuts, hazelnuts, almonds, pecans

½ cup carob powder

Liquid to combine – e.g. water, nut/seed milk, fresh coconut water – to desired consistency

Combine everything in a food blender/processor until all are bound together in a big sticky lump. Divide out into small balls and chill in fridge or freezer.

These can be rolled in powder (i.e. hemp protein 50%) or shredded coconut, decorated with gojis and so on. Use your creativity. Add different things like coconut oil/butter, vanilla, cinnamon, bee pollen, a couple of drops of orange/peppermint oil, maca or camu-camu powder for different tastes and effects.

Matt Monarch's Chia 'Rice Pudding'

Matt has been 100% raw vegan for 10 years, since reading Norman Walker's classic *Become Younger*. Matt is the author of *Raw Spirit* and *Raw Success*. He travels worldwide teaching about eating healthily and healing degenerative diseases. He runs the popular store **The Raw Food World**, plus a daily online TV show. To learn more, visit **www.RawSuccess.org**.

Chia seeds are a wonderfully energizing, light, filling food to use in puddings, cookies and cakes.

Here's a simple chia mock "rice pudding" idea (serves one):

4-5 tbsp dry chia seeds

2 cups nut/seed milk of choice (e.g. almond, hemp milk)

2 tbsp lucuma or mesquite powder

pinch of stevia

big pinch of cinnamon powder

cardamom to taste (optional)

In a blender, mix all the ingredients together, except the chia seeds. Pour the mixture out into a bowl, stir in the chia seeds and let them soak up the liquid for at least 10 minutes before eating. You might also like to stir in some goji berries or coconut chips, top with some goji powder, add maca powder or sprinkle with carob powder, before serving. Enjoy.

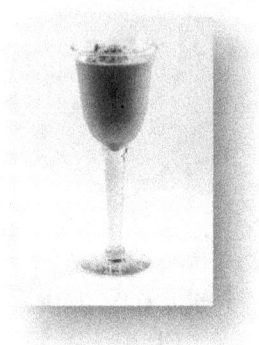

Maria's Heavenly Chocolate Milkshake

A milkshake a day will keep the doctor away! Drink your chocolate!

12 ounces almond milk

1 tbsp raw cacao powder

1 tsp lecithin

1 ½ tbsp pure birch xylitol or other agave nectar

1 tsp vanilla

8 scoops stevia (Trader Joe's pure stevia extract)

1 tsp tocotrienols

½ tsp mucuna pruriens

Celtic or Himalayan salt to taste

1 ½ tsp mesquite pod meal

about 12 – 14 ice cubes

Place all ingredients in blender along with enough ice cubes to give it a "shake" consistency. Blend extra long until smooth and creamy. Enjoy!

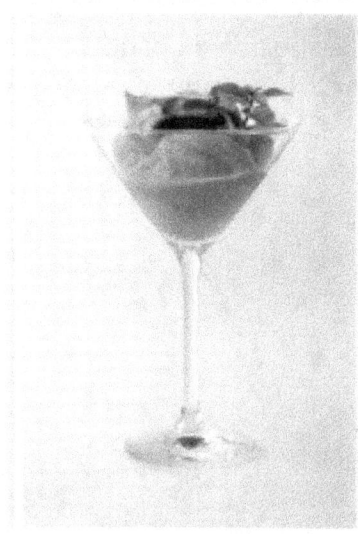

Maria's Strawberry Delight Ice Cream

"Maria's strawberry ice cream is amazing! One night I called Maria, last minute, and asked if she would make me some of her amazing strawberry ice cream (without hesitation she did!) for my daughter's birthday party. My daughter was beyond excited! In fact, everyone enjoyed the strawberry ice cream over the unhealthy chocolate chip cookie dough ice cream cake!" –Cyndi L.

12 ounces almond milk (recipe on page 124 or you can **find the recipe at www.mariarippo.com/recipes**)

2 – 2 ½ large handfuls frozen strawberries or any fruit that sounds fabulous to you!

¼ cup pure birch xylitol, Smart Sweet brand

1 tsp vanilla

8 scoops stevia

Celtic salt to taste

about 12 ice cubes

Place all ingredients into the blender and blend. Continue adding ice cubes until it has an ice cream consistency. Blend on the ice cream setting if your blender has one. Blend until smooth and enjoy immediately. You may freeze any leftover portions.

Almond milk itself is a delectable treat. Simply place two scoops of stevia into a glass and fill the glass with almond milk (recipe on page 124. You may also find my **almond milk recipe online at www.mariarippo.com/blogrecipes.**

Raw Chocolate Pudding

1 avocado

2 tbsp raw cacao powder or organic cocoa powder

2 tbsp agave nectar, maple syrup or honey

⅛ tsp stevia

1 tbsp unrefined coconut oil

1 tsp vanilla

salt to taste

Combine all ingredients in blender and blend until smooth. Enjoy!

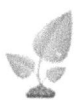

Maria's Hot Fudge

2 tbsp raw cacao

2 tbsp coconut oil

2 tbsp agave nectar, maple syrup or honey

1 tsp vanilla

Celtic or Himalayan salt to taste

Place coconut oil in pan. Heat up on a very low heat just until coconut oil melts. Remove from heat and mix in other ingredients. Pour over strawberry ice cream, swirl in a chocolate shake or just drink it. You may also add this to almond milk (page 124) to make a "to live for" chocolate milk treat for you and your kiddos. Pure bliss.

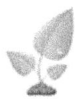

Maria's Raw Chocolate Dream Pie

<u>Crust</u>

1 cup almonds

1 cup walnuts

4 large dates, pitted and chopped

1 tsp vanilla

¼ tsp salt

Combine all ingredients in food processor. Mix until sticky. Press mixture into a greased (with coconut oil) 9" pie plate. Place in freezer or dehydrator for 2 hours to set.

<u>Filling</u>

2 ½ ounces Irish moss: *soak Irish Moss for 4 – 8 hours, then rinse; rinse again to get all of the salt out of it.*

Mix the Irish Moss with 1 cup of water in the blender and blend until very smooth. (The gel will last 2 – 3 weeks in the fridge)

3 tbsp of the Irish Moss mixture

½ cup agave nectar

4 dates, pitted

⅓ cup raw cacao powder

1 ½ cups almond milk (recipe on page 124)

2 tsp vanilla

¼ tsp Celtic or Himalayan salt

2 tbsp ghee

2 tsp tocotrienols (optional)

2 tsp mesquite pod meal (optional)

2 tsp yacon powder (optional)

½ tsp macuna pruriens (optional)

1 ½ cups soaked cashews: *soaked for 4 – 6 hours, drained and rinsed*

7 scoops stevia

Combine above ingredients in blender and blend until very smooth, like pudding. Place in raw pie shell and refrigerate. Enjoy in complete chocolate ecstasy!

IN CLOSING

It is my most sincere desire that The Green Smoothie Challenge will allow you to experience the amazing difference that adding healthy, living, green foods to your diet can make in your state of health. If you are one of the many people on the planet that tends to obsess about aging, gaining unwanted pounds, or falling ill, I hope you feel that you have found a way to alleviate those fears and begin on a new adventure towards total health. Anytime you begin to feel out of control with your eating, simply take The Challenge and get right back on track. You can also do this before a special event or to get ready for a vacation. It is simple to do one day a week, one week a month or ten days a few times a year. Find what works best for you, and go for it.

Cheers to your Wellth!

Maria Rippo

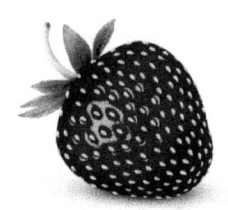

What Will

Your

Story Be?

LINKS

www.mariarippo.com

www.greensmoothiechallenge.com

www.amazon.com

www.bodyecology.com

www.detoxtheworld.com

www.therawfoodworld.com

www.transformationaloils.marketingscents.com

www.wisdomwithinpublishing.com

www.youtube.com/greensmoothiecleanse